live PAIN·FREE

ELIMINATE CHRONIC PAIN WITHOUT DRUGS OR SURGERY

live PAIN-FREE

second edition

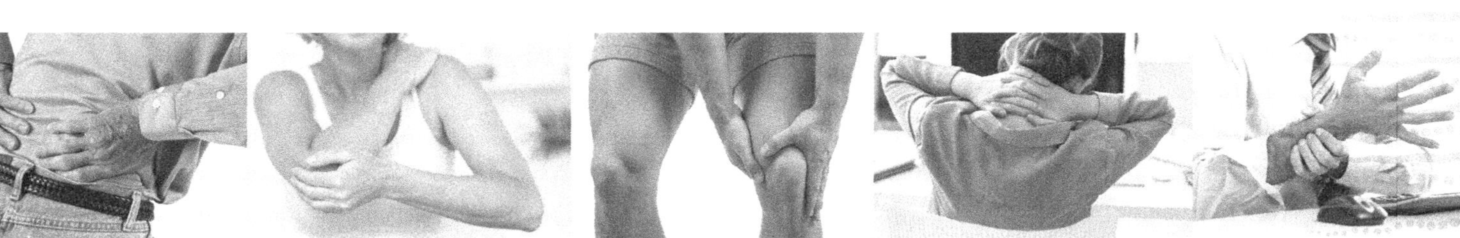

LEE ALBERT, NMT

BESTSELLING AUTHOR OF *YOGA FOR PAIN RELIEF*

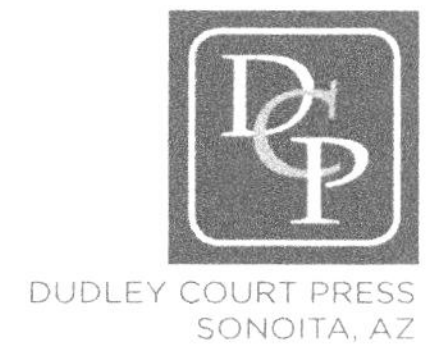

DUDLEY COURT PRESS
SONOITA, AZ

Dudley Court Press
PO Box 102
Sonoita, AZ 85637
www.DudleyCourtPress.com

Connect with Lee Albert at http://www.leealbert.com/
Look for Lee's popular book, *Yoga for Pain Relief,* featured on PBS

Cover and interior design by Dunn+Associates, www.Dunn-Design.com

ISBN paperback: 9781940013497
ISBN ebook 9781940013503
LCCN: 2017958187

Name: Albert, Lee (Lee Michael), 1951-
Title: Live Pain-free : eliminate chronic pain without drugs or surgery / Lee Albert, NMT.
Descriptions: Second edition. | Sonoita, AZ : Dudley Court Press, [2018] | Includes index.
Identifiers: ISBN: 9781940013497 (print) |
Subjects: LCSH: Chronic pain—Alternative treatment. | Chronic pain—Exercise therapy. | Headache— Treatment. | Neck pain—Treatment. | Shoulder pain—Exercise therapy. Backache—Treatment. | Knee—Care and hygiene. | Carpal tunnel syndrome—Treatment. | Fibromyalgia Alternative treatment. | Temporomandibular joint—Diseases—Alternative treatment. Sciatica—Treatment. | Thoracic outlet syndrome—Treatment. | Physical therapy. | Massage therapy. | Self-care, Health.

BISAC: HEALTH & FITNESS / Pain management.
Classification: LCC: RB127 .A397 2018 | DDC: 616/.0472—dc23

Published in the United States of America

To my wife Marcia for her love, support,
encouragement, and editorial advice

To my publisher Gail for her expertise,
dedication, and endless hours of changes

To all my clients and students
who have taught me so much

5-star reviews on Amazon for *Live Pain-free*

I'm a 56 yr. old former elite athlete and currently an avid cyclist. Neck and leg pain was unbearable until I applied Integrated Positional Therapy from this book. It seems counter-intuitive and counter to all PT I've had, but it's practical and works.

—Mary Beall Adler

I work with clients all the time who have pain and this is definitely another good resource. The wrist exercise alone has helped more than twenty of my friends and clients end the wrist pain that they had previously been convinced was "age related" and that they'd have to live with it. Not True! I highly recommend it for practitioners like myself as well as the average person who wants to heal themselves naturally.

—Kathleen Casey

This is an excellent resource. Of particular help is the section on realigning the pelvis. I personally have had some low back issues L-4 and L-5 misalignment/arthritis and some spinal stenosis. By religiously doing these exercises I have avoided surgery so far! I am a yoga teacher and personal trainer and have found the stretches, techniques and suggestions very helpful for my classes and clients.

—Prana gal

Very empowering to be able to take care of some things without consulting a healthcare professional! Buy this book! We admire the efficacy and simple wisdom of his suggestions. Clearly, the man knows what he is talking about.

—Samyel Fon

The easy exercises in this book have greatly reduced my chronic lower back pain. I would recommend this book for anyone who experiences pain and wants to take as few drugs as possible.

—Movie Maven

The book is easy to follow and puts all Lee Albert's teachings in one place. It is a fantastic reference tool and I highly recommend it.

—Kctco

Excellent bodywork routine! —David Leung

This is a wonderful book. I used the sequence for low back pain and it worked right away. More people need to know about this. —Cryogini

I am using the postures for the neck and find them to be practical and effective. I would recommend this product to anyone who is ready to become responsible for maintaining the physical body without drugs or surgery as the title suggests.
—Clara Frazier

This is another very good resource for those who want to take a more active role in obtaining and maintaining their health. The techniques in this book are helpful and useful. Ongoing pain has given me a run for the money. I hate taking meds. This is a tool to educate and help yourself. —Lynn Ruediger

In very easy to understand terms the author explains how to counter the many aches and pains our ordinary and sedentary life styles cause. —Kathy

This book has saved my back more than once. I've lent it out to friends with back issues and pregnant friends who also found it helped immensely. And I've given it as a gift to family members with back and pain issues. It's nothing short of miraculous. —Lisa Tener

contents

foreword to the second edition 13
foreword to the first edition 17
introduction 21

chapter 1: muscle imbalances: the key to unlocking pain 23
chapter 2: what's your pain problem?
symptoms and conditions check-in 31
chapter 3: overview of integrated positional therapy (IPT) wellness plans 35
chapter 4: IPT wellness plan for tension-type headaches and migraines 41
chapter 5: IPT wellness plan for temporomandibular joint disorder (TMJ)...... 49
chapter 6: IPT wellness plan for cervical muscle strain (neck pain) 55
chapter 7: IPT wellness plan for thoracic outlet syndrome (TOS) 61
chapter 8: IPT wellness plan for thoracic muscle strain (upper back pain) 67
chapter 9: IPT wellness plan for epicondylitis, lateral or medial
(tennis or golfer's elbow 73
chapter 10: IPT wellness plan for carpal tunnel syndrome (CTS) 79
chapter 11: IPT wellness plan for hip pain (bursitis) 85
chapter 12: IPT wellness plan for lumbar muscle strain (low back pain) 91
chapter 13: IPT wellness plan for piriformis syndrome (sciatica) 97
chapter 14: IPT wellness plan for medial meniscus injury (knee pain) 103
chapter 15: IPT wellness plan for plantar fasciitis (heel spur) 109
chapter 16: IPT wellness plan for fibromyalgia 115
chapter 17: the basic care of your body 121

thank you 127

acknowledgments 129

caution 131

appendix a: proper sitting, driving, and computer positions 134

appendix b: four stretches to balance the pelvis 137

appendix c: three neck stretches 141

appendix d: jaw 143

appendix e: shoulders 144

appendix f: chest exercises 146

appendix g: arm and hand exercises 147

appendix h: hip and buttocks exercises 149

appendix i: inner thigh exercises 150

appendix j: lower leg exercises 151

index 153

about the author 159

We stand, sit, and walk every day.
If you can improve your alignment and efficiency
in these activities, you will go a long way
in reducing your pain.

—Ingrid Bacci, PhD

foreword
to the second edition

I'm delighted, honored, and humbled to write this foreword to Lee Albert's beloved book, *Live Pain-free: Eliminate Chronic Pain without Drugs or Surgery.* Thousands of us waited impatiently for this important work to arrive on the bookshelves. When it did, I can joyfully attest it was worth the wait. This book is overflowing with wonderful, profound, simple (and simply profound) tools and techniques for self-healing. Lee Albert has been my go-to healer for twenty years.

I do not use the word "healer" lightly. When Lee first arrived in the Healing Arts Department at Kripalu Center, where I have been a longtime faculty member, he soon became renowned as a miracle worker. Having been around the spiritual and holistic health world for so long, I was not only skeptical, I actually rolled my eyes. I had seen hundreds of teachers, gurus, and self-professed "healers" come and go. Some of them had accompanying bad behavior to add fuel to my irritated fire. I want my teachers to walk their talk. In my world, permission to be human is granted, but permission to be arrogant and awful is not. Through the years, I had spent a lot of money on bodyworkers who bragged they knew exactly what was wrong with me and would cure all. Dancing and teaching yoga on thinly disguised concrete floors for decades had created all kinds of foot, knee, and hip and back issues in my valiant body.

Eventually, with a rueful sigh, I signed up for this new Integrated Positional Therapy modality to see what all the excitement was about. I doubted this man would accomplish much, but with a shrug, I marched up to the fourth floor where this stranger, Lee Albert, was waiting.

Wow. Was I ever wrong. I met a mild-mannered, laid back, kind, easy-going, "normal" guy who explained that with Integrated Positional Therapy nothing should hurt, and that I would feel better quickly. Still skeptical, I told him about my meniscus issues, my unhappy knees, and how challenging it was to direct my own Let Your Yoga Dance Teacher Training, as well as Yoga Teacher Training, while limping! He promised that all would be well.

Lee proceeded to offer some simple techniques: balancing my hips, finding trigger spots where the pain dwelled, working his magic. In one hour, I got off that table feeling ever so much better. I still had a ways to go with my meniscus issue, and Lee gave me some excellent self-help homework to keep me on track. Before saying good-bye, he shared, with a twinkle in his eye, his most important assignment. "Now go right down to the Kripalu Shop and get yourself some dark chocolate." Although I don't eat chocolate, his assignment made me laugh. And my body felt great. I thought: Now this guy is the real deal!

Twenty years later, my knees are still doing well; they still dance and teach on disguised concrete! No surgery. No crutches. Just occasional tune-up sessions and ongoing self-care.

Lee has helped me through all my set backs, realigning my body to equanimity and balance again and again. He helped me heal my ongoing neck issues by sharing a foolproof neck stretch (found in Appendix C of this book). Not only do I use this technique for myself, I offer it to my students in yoga class.

In 2012, while on retreat visiting a serene, bucolic abbey, I discovered that the Mother Abbess had been suffering for months with severe neck pain. I explained that although Integrated Positional Therapy was not my day job, I might be able to help her. She lay down on a mat, and I used Lee's neck stretches. Thirty minutes later she was pain-free, bowing to me, calling me a worker of miracles! I laughed and told her all about Lee. "Might I buy his book?" she begged.

As the years rolled by, Lee and I became pals and colleagues at Kripalu Center. We started a race to see who could write their book most quickly. He won by two years, and then became my cheerleader to get mine on the bookshelves. Whenever we see each other in the halls of Kripalu, we exchange hugs and high fives.

At last, Lee's second book arrived in June of 2017, much to the delight of the yoga community: Yoga for Pain Relief. Long ago Lee transformed the way I practice and teach yoga. His knowledge, respect, and love for the human body is vast; he imparts this knowledge so simply that it becomes fun and easy to grasp for this humanities and fine arts brain.

Teaching and training thousands of people a year at Kripalu and elsewhere, I am in a position to offer advice. Whenever my students complained of ongoing physical issues, I used to say: "Make an appointment with Lee." And then I would watch that student return to class later on with a twinkle in the eye and a new body. Every single time. Nowadays, due to popular demand, it is not as easy to get a session with Lee. But the good news is that now you can get an Integrated Positional Therapy session because Lee has trained many others in the healing arts department. I did manage to get my skeptical older brother, Peter, a session due to his newly replaced hip. Lee helped him tremendously. Peter was thrilled and continues his exercises on a daily basis. Lee has trained hundreds of bodyworkers, yogis, and lovers of the body who flock to his programs and trainings. He does not give us fish; he teaches us how to fish.

Lee often says: "Your body is always trying to heal itself. All you have to do is learn how to listen to it. The body has great wisdom. Whenever your body is telling you one thing and your brain is telling you something else, always listen to the body. The brain can make up some pretty good stories that are not necessarily true" (*Live Pain-free*).

I truly love this book, *Live Pain-free;* the pictures are clear and the content excellent. Wherever pain might dwell in the body, Lee has a good solution, with accompanying homework to keep that body part healthy. Lee's gentle, kind, loving spirit comes through each page.

As a teacher and trainer, I have placed both *Live Pain-free and Yoga for Pain Relief* on my required reading lists for all my students and trainees. As a practitioner, I refer to them often.

I am forever grateful to Lee for giving me (and the world) a great gift: a surefire way to heal the body. You are lucky to be holding this book in your hands. And it is written by someone who is just as wise and wonderful as the words you are about to read. Enjoy the book and your new body!

A Lee-loving chocolate hug to you,
Megha Nancy Buttenheim, MA / E-RYT 1000
CEO, CJO (Chief JOY Officer) and Founding Director: Let Your Yoga Dance®
Author of Expanding Joy: Let Your Yoga Dance, Embodying Positive Psychology

foreword
to the first edition

You and your body are healing geniuses. Let me show you all the ways.

Pain definitely gets my attention, and I love finding easy, natural solutions for pain relief and, whenever possible of course, elimination of pain.

I'm writing the foreword for this book because I know, through my own physical experience of pain and the absence of pain, that this system—Integrated Positional Therapy—really works. Here's how it worked and continues to work for me!

Some years ago I started a dance practice. After awhile, I developed some heel pain which then worsened, and I started limping because of it. I visited a chiropractor for months, which helped a little, but the pain continued. Acupuncture didn't significantly help either.

I started a new stretching regime, but when the pain continued with no relief I visited an orthopedic doctor who treats the dancers in the San Francisco ballet. She watched me walk and diagnosed plantar fasciitis. She recommended orthotics, which I started using. Those didn't help either.

I then bought a portable laser device and also began icing my heels after every walk I took. I'm a daily walker and began walking shorter and shorter distances due to the unresolved pain.

It was all very disheartening and I felt hopeless. My health was being compromised from my lack of mobility.

That's when I met Lee Albert, NMT, at Kripalu, and experienced Integrated Positional Therapy for the first time.

In the session, I warned Lee that if he squeezed my heels, the pain was so acute that I might be tempted to punch him.

He smiled gently and said, "I can show you how to resolve that in about ninety seconds."

I felt very skeptical but also drawn to his mild mannered, ego-less approach.

As he moved my body into various gentle positions, I couldn't imagine how this could be effective all.

Then he showed me how to gently bend my foot backward and hold the position. I felt tempted to push the position further for "greater benefit," and he said simply, "This is not like stretching."

He then said, "I'm like a carpenter. My job is to show you how to be plumb, level, and straight. If you like how you feel, you'll do your homework."

Then he squeezed my heel and rotated my foot.

I waited for the cascade of pain and felt vague, faraway remnants of the memory of a pain. I looked at him and absolutely marveled.

He said, "It will take about ten days to two weeks to reset the muscle memory completely so you have no pain."

Now I was very eager to see how this same principle might work for the rest of my body!

As Lee worked and showed me various positions, he said, "I'll be giving you handouts so that you'll have the visuals to practice with and do your homework. I'm here to show you how to do this for yourself."

I immediately doubted that I could do it without him and said so.

He replied, "This is not a system where you need me. All you need is yourself, your body, and the willingness to practice." Then he added, "Old people are not bent over or crooked because they're old. They're that way because they've been crooked longer."

This statement and the system made practical sense to me, but I wasn't experiencing the dramatic release of pain in other parts of my body like I had with my heels.

Until I got up off the table.

I had a sensation of what I remember about being seven years old, and realized that it was complete freedom from pain. Even though I had very minor, nondebilitating pain in the rest of my body, I didn't realize how it might feel to be without it.

It felt utterly transformative and releasing, and I felt like skipping.

Lee patiently explained that I had homework to do, and showed me the handouts and explained the main positions. I left his office clutching the papers and grinning at my good fortune.

Then I skipped across the wildflower meadow and felt like a commercial for this system. I wanted to call Oprah and everyone else with a giant audience and say, "Let's show this to *everybody*!"

Of course I also wanted to share the system with all of my readers too, but there wasn't a book or DVD yet.

I of course told my friends and family and showed them how to do specific positions. I experienced incredible changes in my neck, shoulders, and hips, and reveled in feeling pain-free in new ways; I continued practicing.

I also showed people I didn't know, like the guy who sold me my new car who limped over to hand me the contract. I knew immediately what he had. When I asked him why he was limping, he said: "Yeah, the doctor says plantar fasciitis, and I'm also older and heavier, so it's bound to happen."

I showed him the ninety-second hold for each foot and gave an abbreviated description of Integrated Positional Therapy.

The next day, I returned to pick up my new car, and this man ran toward me, shouting, "No pain! No pain! No limping! My God! It really works!" He hugged me and asked if there was a book about it so he could learn more. I assured him that one day there would be.

I loved the simple, practical, do-it-myself aspect of this new system and began to do my homework daily.

It was immediately clear, and just as Lee had said, when I did the homework, my body felt better. When I didn't, the aches and pains returned.

I mostly did the homework—which is about five minutes a day—and felt better.

Each year when I returned to teach at Kripalu, I made an appointment to see Lee and learn even more about the system. I also wished for a teacher in San Francisco where I lived to periodically show me more nuances and sometimes work with me too. I knew that Lee trained people in this system, but so far I hadn't found anybody else who knew it.

I also wished for a book or a DVD that I could use at home to expand my practice.

I could see that Lee was so occupied showing people how to do Integrated Positional Therapy that he didn't necessarily have the time or energy to create a book or DVD.

I decided to share that I was an author and would do anything I could to help him publish his book, including write an endorsement or foreword, which he enthusiastically responded to and confirmed my thoughts about his time and energy for creating a book or DVD.

Then the day came when Lee told me that he was working with a publisher on the book!

I prayed that he'd met somebody good that would help him.

And he had.

That's how this foreword came to be, and now you can experience this system for yourself and share it with others, too.

Our bodies are truly miraculous healing devices if we just know the right buttons and knobs and if we know the Integrated Positional Release system.

And now you will too.

Happy practicing and living without pain!

With love, Susan (aka SARK)
Author, Artist, Succulent Wild Woman
http://www.PlanetSARK.com

introduction

as this second edition of *Live Pain-free* goes to press, I look back at the impact that the first edition has had and am so grateful. I have received numerous emails from my readers expressing their gratitude for my book and the pain relief it has given them. I'm about to film a PBS show with Peggy Cappy that will demonstrate to a large audience the root causes of pain and how to remedy it. This book has changed the way people think about their pain and has given them hope that they, too, can live pain-free by practicing these easy exercises. For those who don't know how this started, let me share the story.

On a beautiful summer day, the shining sun felt wonderful on my skin. I had recently completed my studies to be a massage therapist. Driving along the highways of the placid Quebec countryside, I slowly pushed on the brake to stop at a stop sign. Suddenly in my rearview mirror I saw a car racing toward me. I knew right away that it wouldn't stop. Smack! I was rear-ended at 60 mph.

Fortunately I was wearing my seat belt and didn't hit my head on the windshield. I got out of the car, which was a total wreck. I couldn't believe it. I was fine—nothing broken or bleeding, which was a miracle.

Pretty soon the police came along. When they asked how I was doing, I said I was a little shaken up but thought I was fine. Due to the severity of the crash, the officer insisted I go the emergency room to have a doctor look me over. At the hospital, a doctor checked my vital signs, did a few range-of-motion tests for my neck, and said he thought I would be fine.

And I was fine . . . for three weeks. Then I started to get migraine headaches. I'd had headaches before, but never a migraine. These were excruciating! External smells, sounds, or bright lights would set them off. I could barely stand it. My doctor decided I should start physical therapy. Little did I know that I was going to have these headaches once a week for the next three years.

I spent those three years visiting nearly every therapist I could find. I was desperate for relief. I spent tens of thousands of dollars and sought out the best therapies I could find—all with no results. Then one day my whole life changed.

I went to a highly recommended therapist who did gentle forms of therapy that didn't seem like they were going to help much. After the session, I thanked her and headed home, disappointed, knowing this wasn't going to work any more than all the other therapies I had tried.

Much to my surprise, however, the migraine headaches never returned. How could this be? One session, no deep work, and my headaches were gone? Impossible! I had tried almost every kind of therapy I could think of and nothing had worked. How could this gentle, simple therapy do the trick in one short therapy session and relieve the horrendous pain I'd been suffering with for over three years?

I set out on a quest to find out what this therapy was and how it worked. I wanted to know and to share it with everyone on the planet.

This book is a result of my quest. I've been practicing and teaching Integrated Positional Therapy now for thirty-plus years, helping thousands of people to enjoy permanent pain relief without surgery or drugs. I hope this book will help you and your loved ones find relief from painful conditions with gentle therapeutic techniques and simple, ongoing self-care.

A quick note here to those readers who tend to go directly to their particular condition: I appreciate your enthusiasm, but you will benefit most by reading the first three chapters and the last chapter before jumping to your condition. There is important information in those chapters that will be most beneficial in your quest to feel better. One of the most important things you will learn will be how to stretch. Stretching incorrectly can lead to poor results or can aggravate your pain.

As this work continues to become better known, I am excited to report that I have an ongoing certification program. Currently we have nineteen certified practitioners and more on the way. These practitioners have completed a comprehensive training program, and I am grateful for their dedication, commitment, and caring. I am delighted to have their assistance in teaching people to be pain-free. If you are in need of a practitioner, please visit my website (www.LeeAlbert.com). My goal is to have a grassroots movement and create a village where an educated populace can treat themselves for many of their aches and pains, thus reducing the costs of health care. With your help, this is possible! Together we do make a difference!

Lee Albert
www.LeeAlbert.com
Lenox, Massachusetts

CHAPTER 1

muscle imbalances: the key to unlocking pain

Pain! Everyone experiences pain at some point. The problem of chronic pain in our bodies is complex and far-reaching. Musculoskeletal pain encompasses many different areas, such as the head, neck, back, limbs, joints, bones, and even chronic, nonspecific, widespread tissue pain.

At least one hundred million Americans suffer from chronic pain. Chronic pain is defined as pain lasting longer than six months. That number goes much higher when we add the statistics for acute pain. Chronic and acute pain can range from mild to moderate to excruciating. According to a recent Institute of Medicine Report: *Relieving Pain in America: A Blueprint for Transforming Prevention, Care, Education, and Research,* pain is a significant public health problem that costs society at least $560–$635 billion annually.

Pain is a huge economic burden both on our health care system and on individuals. Not only does it cause higher insurance rates, but it also creates various additional financial costs for the individual. Studies have shown that individuals with acute or chronic pain have much higher out-of-pocket expenses, therefore leaving less money for other necessities that we deem important (like . . . having a lot more fun!). Employers are also impacted because of lost workdays, as adults with pain report missing more days from work than people without pain. Chronic pain affects more people than the combined dollars spent for cancer, heart disease, and diabetes.

Despite the wide-ranging conditions and symptoms, all types of musculoskeletal pain share similar underlying mechanisms, manifestations, and potential treatments. In the final analysis, most pain is foundational, resulting from imbalances in a musculoskeletal system that is out of alignment. A great deal of research presents evidence that the root cause of many neuromuscular pain patterns is due to biomechanical misalignments caused by muscle imbalances. We are in pain because we are misaligned, or "crooked." Therapists often refer to this as the muscles being "locked long" or "locked short."

Remember when your mother told you to sit up or stand up straight? Well, she was right! Your mother probably didn't know it at the time, but good posture is more than simply about looking good. Good posture is essential to a healthy, functioning, pain-free body. Most of your pain is caused by poor posture. You are in pain because you are misaligned or . . . crooked! Even if you think you have good posture, you probably don't. Many misalignments are not obvious to the untrained eye.

This may seem too simple, but let's look at some examples. Picture a house in your mind. Imagine that the basement of the house is a little lower on one side. In other words, the house is crooked. Over time, the crooked house develops all sorts of structural problems, i.e. the roof might leak, windows are hard to open, the chimney leans, etc. The structure of the building is not carrying the load the way it was designed because it is not straight. All these problems are caused by one condition: the house is crooked.

You could also imagine a car with its front end out of alignment. The car will run, but the tires will have abnormal strain on them because the car is crooked, and those tires will wear out more quickly than if they were aligned.

The solution in each case is to bring the building or the car back into proper alignment—give the car or the building "good posture" so it carries its load the way it was designed to.

Let's apply this theory to the human body and your pain. Do you know what the following conditions have in common: sciatica, plantar fasciitis, carpal tunnel, tennis elbow, low back pain, neck pain, and most headaches?

At first, they don't seem to have much in common. They occur in different parts of the body and involve different musculoskeletal structures. However, if you step back and look at the body as a whole, you will notice the common element.

This common element is called **muscle imbalance**. This simply means that some muscles are too short and some muscles are too long. Both muscles will feel tight. The short muscle is contracted and tight, and the long muscle is like an overstretched rubber band—too long and very tight.

Since every muscle is attached to a bone, these muscle imbalances pull the bones out of alignment. That's what makes you crooked.

Optimal functioning of the musculoskeletal system requires that muscles be in balance in regard to strength and length. If they do not possess this balance, then the muscles become painful and the joint where these imbalances are occurring will become compromised. This often manifests as pain in that joint and/or limited range of motion.

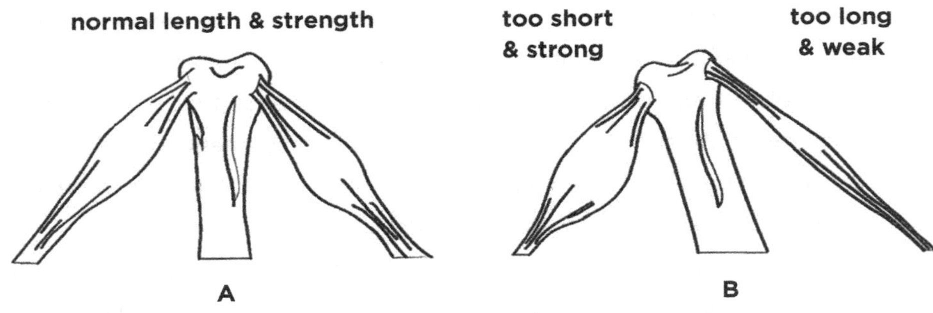

Illustration A demonstrates what muscles in balance look like. They are equal in both length and strength. Illustration B demonstrates what a muscle imbalance looks like. Notice that the muscle on the left in Illustration B is short and contracted. (This muscle is then considered strong.) The muscle on the right in Illustration B is too long and overstretched. (This muscle is then considered weak.) These small imbalances will cause the bigger imbalances we see in the next diagram.

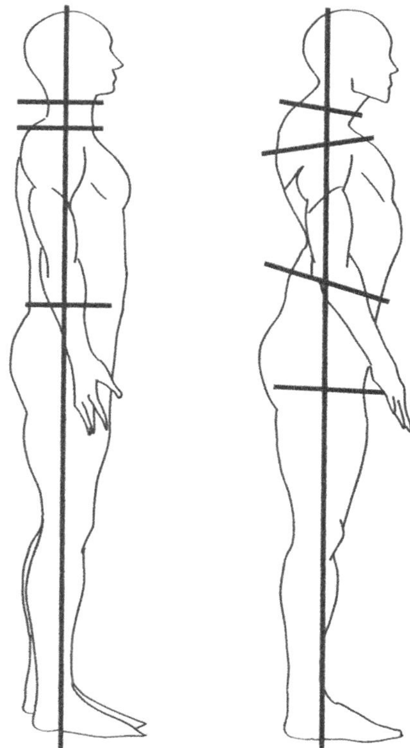

The figure on the left is what a balanced body looks like. The figure on the right has numerous muscle imbalances. Most people exhibit at least some of these imbalances and are not even aware that they have muscle imbalances. Another way to think about imbalances is to look at your posture. If you have poor posture, you have muscle imbalances like the figure on the right. If your muscles are in balance, you have good posture like the figure on the left. To be concise, a muscle imbalance is when some muscles are too short and tight, and some muscles are too long and tight.

Misalignment of the skeletal structure caused by muscle imbalance can cause compressions of the nerves, discs, and other structures in the body. It can also cause the fascia to be twisted. Fascia is a band of fibrous connective tissue enveloping, separating, or binding together muscles, organs, and other soft structures of the body. These twists, compressions, and tight muscles ultimately lead to less oxygen in the tissues at those areas. The medical term for this condition is ischemia, which means an inadequate supply of blood is reaching the tissues. As a result, the tissue is not getting enough oxygen. **That lack of oxygen is what causes a good deal of the pain.**

We all have demands that keep us working through our pain. So we continually re-strain the same muscles through our daily activities until we learn how to do those activities without causing muscle strain. The protocols listed in this book will help you perform your daily activities with no pain or show you how to relieve the pain that occurs because of these activities. Our plan is to reduce or eliminate as many causes of muscle strain as we can and apply stretches or slackenings (I discuss slackening in detail in chapter 3) to correct the muscle imbalances.

One of the most common causes of these muscle imbalances is simply poor posture and/or improper ergonomics. Slumping at your desk or in your car pushes your head forward of your body, putting a lot of strain on your neck and shoulders, which now have to hold up your head without the support of the spinal column. The average head weighs between eight and twelve pounds. That is very heavy. If you tried to hold that much weight with your arms, you probably would not last more than five minutes. Yet we ask our neck and shoulder muscles to hold that weight all day long. These muscles are not designed to hold up your head. They are meant to move your head in different directions, not hold them in the same position for long periods of time. By correcting your computer and driving positions, you will bring your head over your shoulders and improve your posture. Your bones (the spinal column) will be holding up your head, which will help take the strain off the muscles.

To summarize, muscle imbalances pull the frame of the body (the bones) into misalignment, causing pain in the body. The condition of being out of alignment or crooked results in many neuromuscular pain patterns. An estimated 80% of all the pain you will experience in your life is due to these misaligned mechanical problems. Muscles that are either too long or too short pull your bones crooked, causing compression and reducing oxygen to the tissues.

The key to understanding and eliminating pain is to be able to recognize the cause. When you go to a doctor, you could be diagnosed with any one of hundreds of conditions. In our Western model of medicine, standard treatment for conditions like sciatica, plantar fasciitis, carpal tunnel, tennis elbow, low back pain, neck pain, and most headaches involves treating the symptoms, typically with a painkiller, an anti-inflammatory drug, or sometimes even surgery. Seldom does treatment address the cause. The cause is muscle imbalance or misalignment, and the correct treatment is to get you "uncrooked."

muscles develop imbalances due to over or underuse

In our daily lives, we have all developed habits that impact our muscular system. These habits are things we usually do every day in our jobs, such as the way we sit and what we choose for exercise or don't choose for exercise. All of our daily actions require that we use or don't use our muscles in a particular way. Some of our muscles we use a lot and some we use far less.

Since all muscles are attached to bones and other connective tissue, providing skeletal stability and support, muscle imbalances due to muscle tension, trauma, repetitive, or improper use can lead to excessive muscle shortening or lengthening—allowing for the movement of skeletal components that create postural misalignments, musculoskeletal stresses, and pain. In short, the root cause is muscular imbalances. In simple terms, some muscles become too long and some muscles become too short, leading to postural distortions and pain. As the imbalance becomes greater, the individual experiences pain that becomes more severe.

The muscles we use often will tend to get shorter and stronger. The muscles we use less often tend to get longer and weaker. The way we sit also puts some muscles in a contracted position and some in a more extended position often for long periods of time. For example, when you are slumping in a chair, you will notice that the chest muscles have become shorter and the muscles between your shoulder blades (rhomboids) have become longer.

Finally, we are going to talk about the solution to your muscle imbalances and your aches and pains.

integrated positional therapy to the rescue

Integrated Positional Therapy teaches you how to quickly identify the most common misalignments and to develop a quick and simple approach to getting back into balance. IPT is a gentle and simple self-care approach that has been shown to be effective at successfully addressing a wide range of common acute/chronic neuromuscular conditions and associative pain. Unlike conventional treatment methods that focus on the symptoms of pain and pain management, IPT takes a novel approach to eliminate neuromuscular pain at its root cause.

With a focus on the close relationship that musculoskeletal imbalances play in the development of general and localized pain, IPT delivers simple, therapeutic self-care techniques that anyone can do. These techniques help identify and correct muscular imbalances and effectively hone in on many of the root causes of pain. This pain relief may be achieved with strengthening and stretching exercises or targeted yoga poses.

Integrated Positional Therapy (IPT) is based upon the osteopathic techniques of strain/counterstrain and muscle energy technique. Strain/counterstrain slackens a muscle and makes it shorter, while muscle energy technique stretches a muscle and makes it longer.

Please don't be concerned about the technical terms. These techniques are simply used to bring your body back into alignment and out of pain gently and quickly. Muscle energy technique (MET) and strain/counterstrain are used to correct the imbalances in the muscles.

MET is a powerful tool to quickly and easily lengthen tight, constricted muscles and restore range of motion. It is a form of stretching using active isometric contractions.

Strain/counterstrain can also be applied to these tight, constricted muscles. With this technique, the affected area is passively shortened and held for two minutes, thereby allowing the muscle fibers to effectively reset and return to neutral. The results are often dramatic and long lasting.

One of the first principles therapists and doctors learn is that the body, including the musculoskeletal system, is always trying to achieve homeostasis. This means that it is trying to get back into balance or alignment. The great thing is that we are doing this every day, but it's something we are not usually aware of. Here's an example. Do you ever lie down on your back and instinctively put your hands under your head? You probably don't think about the movement consciously. You do it because it feels good; your body automatically does it. Why? Because your body is trying to get back into balance. This movement of putting your hands under your head releases and rebalances the shoulders and part of the neck.

Try this experiment for yourself:

Place your left hand on your right shoulder. If you are wearing a shirt you might find a seam in the shirt in this area. With your left hand press somewhere along the seam. This will be tender or sore in many people. Once you have found a tender spot, take your right arm and gently rest the forearm on top of your head. Now press the spot that was sore before. Does it feel better? It usually does. Now hold your right arm in this position on top of your head for two minutes. This period allows the muscle memory to reset. After two minutes, put your right arm back down at your side. Press the tender spot again. It should feel better. The effects of this technique are cumulative, so each time the pain gets lesser and lesser.

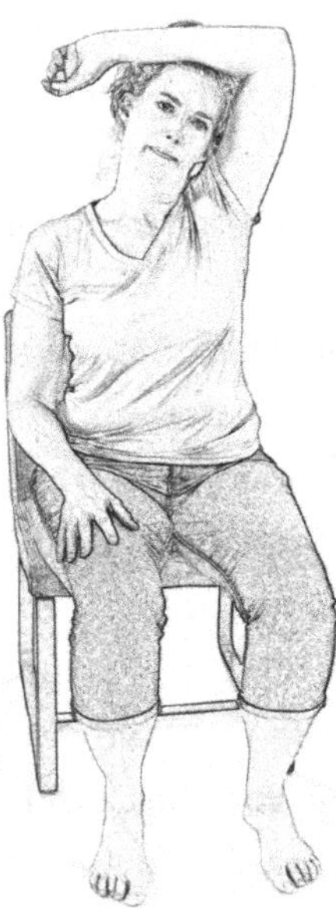

After you have found the sore spot, this is the position of the arm that will relieve the pain.

Here is another example. Do you ever sit in a chair and cross your legs? Almost everyone does this and yet we don't generally think about it. Our body naturally crosses our legs for us because the position feels good. The body is trying to achieve homeostasis or balance by gently stretching the outside of the hip and leg. When your body is in balance, it just plain feels good. (Common wisdom is that crossing your legs while sitting in a chair is bad for you, but it is simply the body's way of stretching the muscles on the outside of the leg and hip to bring them back into balance.) When your muscles are in balance, you will no longer cross your legs because it is not needed.

Your body is always trying to heal itself. All you have to do is learn how to listen to what it is trying to tell you. The body has great wisdom. Whenever your body is telling you one thing and your brain is telling you something else, always listen to the body. The brain can make up some pretty good stories that are not necessarily true.

Positional Therapy is the therapy that alleviated my migraines. I developed Integrated Positional Therapy (IPT) by adding critical components to make the therapy even more effective in relieving chronic pain. IPT is what I now practice and want to share with you in this book. In addition to the basic muscle release techniques of Positional Therapy, Integrated Positional Therapy includes important exercises to straighten the pelvis and adds Wellness Plans to enhance the immediate and long-term results.

Integrated Positional Therapy (IPT) is designed to eliminate pain at its root cause and not to simply hide the symptoms. As a self-care technique, this therapy can help you to correct the muscle imbalances in your own body.

With some easy-to-learn practices, you will learn to correct the imbalances by making your short muscles longer and your long muscles shorter. This process will often bring your body into alignment and out of pain.

IPT can eliminate or reduce the pain associated with many common conditions, such as headaches and migraines, back and neck pain, carpal tunnel syndrome, limited range of motion and sports injuries, thoracic outlet syndrome, sciatica, repetitive motion injuries, fibromyalgia, tendonitis, plantar fasciitis, and many more. This book covers thirteen of the most common conditions. In some cases, a session with a trained Integrated Positional Therapist may be advisable, but most people will find great relief from chronic muscle pain by following the appropriate Wellness Plan described in this book.

Simple, easy-to-do-at-home exercises and other lifestyle habits will maintain the results. Ongoing maintenance is crucial to keeping your body pain-free. Remember the car analogy? Just as your car needs regular maintenance to stay in great working order, your body requires maintenance to stay pain-free. Just fifteen to twenty minutes a day is often all that is required.

The treatment protocols described in this manual are based upon thirty-plus years of clinical experience treating tens of thousands of people with superior results. In the pages that follow, you will learn how to correct your own muscle imbalances. You will learn exactly what is causing your pain. You'll learn how to improve the quality of your life by reducing or eliminating the pain in your body that you are currently enduring. You will also learn some general tips on how to be healthier. Everything I am going to show you is easy and takes little time to do. No previous experience is needed. No special equipment is necessary. These practices are designed to fit your busy lifestyle. As a matter of fact, many of the practices can be done in bed, on the couch, or at the office.

So let's get started!

CHAPTER 2

what's your pain problem?

symptoms and conditions check-in

Check the following chart to find the condition that most closely describes your symptoms. It does not need to be a perfect match.

Test for the condition until you confirm which condition is creating your symptoms. If none of the tests confirm a particular condition, choose the Wellness Plan for the condition that is most closely associated with your symptoms. If you have several conditions, choose the Wellness Plan for the dominant or primary condition to start.

If these are your symptoms	You may suffer from	Do this test to confirm
Sensation of pain, tightness, or pressure around the forehead or back of the head and neck. The pain is sometimes described as throbbing or aching and can affect the front, top, or side of the head.	Tension-Type Headaches and Migraines	No test is necessary. If you have persistent headaches, see your health care provider, as this could be a sign of a more serious problem.
Sensation of pain or tightness in the jaw or in front of the ear with sounds, such as clicking, grating, and/or popping. Can also cause headaches and earaches and make it difficult to open your mouth wide.	Temporomandibular Joint Disorder (TMJ)	With the mouth open, press lightly on the joint near the ear. If this is painful, this could be TMJ or tight, sore muscles that could be a precursor to the condition. If you cannot open your mouth very wide or it is painful to do so, this could be also be TMJ.

If these are your symptoms	You may suffer from	Do this test to confirm
Sensation of pain in the neck that could be described as an ache, stiffness, burning, or stabbing. This condition can be acute or chronic. It is often better in certain positions such as lying down or standing.	Cervical Muscle Strain (Neck Pain)	Bend your head in different directions. If you feel pain, stiffness, or aching, this could be neck pain or tight, sore muscles that could be a precursor to the condition.
Sensation of pain, numbness, tingling, weakness, or coldness in the arm and/or hand.	Thoracic Outlet Syndrome (TOS)	Raise both hands over your head with fingers pointing toward the ceiling and palms facing straight ahead. Rapidly open and close hands. Do this for one minute. If you feel numbness, tingling, or coldness within the minute, this could be TOS or tight, sore muscles that could be a precursor to the condition.
Pain in the upper back that is often described as an ache, tightness, burning, or stabbing. This condition can be acute or chronic. It is often better in certain positions, such as lying down or standing or sitting. It is usually worse with long periods of sitting in a chair or reading in bed. The pain may also radiate down the arms.	Thoracic Muscle Strain (Upper Back Pain)	Bend your body in different directions. If you feel pain, stiffness, or aching, this could be upper back pain or tight, sore muscles that could be a precursor to the condition.
Sensation of pain or discomfort at the site of the elbow, sometimes radiating to other parts of the arm. This could be the inside or outside of the elbow.	Epicondylitis, Lateral or Medial (Tennis or Golfer's Elbow)	Hold your right arm out in front of you with elbow straight and palm facing down. With the left hand, bend the right wrist so that the fingers on the right hand are pointing up toward the ceiling. Then bend the right hand at the wrist down toward the floor so the fingers are pointing down. If this causes pain on the outside of the elbow, it could be tennis elbow. If this causes pain on the inside of the elbow, this could be golfer's elbow or tight, sore muscles that could be a precursor to the condition. Test the other side.

If these are your symptoms	**You may suffer from**	**Do this test to confirm**
Sensation of pain, numbness, tingling, burning, or weakness in the hand and fingers.	Carpal Tunnel Syndrome (CTS)	Test for CTS on the right hand. From a normal standing position with your arms at your side, bend your right elbow to 90 degrees with your palm facing down. Use your left hand to gently push your right hand toward the floor, creating a bend in the wrist. If you develop pain, numbness, tingling, burning, or weakness in the hand and fingers within a minute, this could be CTS or tight, sore muscles that could be a precursor to the condition. Test on the other side.
Symptoms can be pain on the outside of the hip or in the groin area. Sometimes this pain originates from the low back. The pain can range from mild to severe. It may be sharp or just a little achy. The pain may make walking difficult. The pain is often worse with activity.	Hip Pain (Bursitis)	Pain in the hip or groin area that is worse when walking or weight bearing.
Sensation of pain in the lower back that could be described as an ache, stiffness, burning, or stabbing. This condition can be acute or chronic. It is often better in certain positions, such as lying down or standing.	Lumbar Muscle Strain (Low Back Pain)	Gently bend your body in different directions. If you feel pain, stiffness, or aching, this could be low back pain or tight, sore muscles that could be a precursor to the condition.
Sensation of pain, numbness, tingling, or weakness that you feel in your back or buttocks and down your leg, which sometimes may move into your foot.	Piriformis Syndrome (Sciatica)	Sit upright on the edge of a chair. Place one ankle on the opposite thigh. Keeping the back straight, bend forward at the waist while bringing your chest toward your knee. If this movement increases the numbness or tingling, this could be piriformis syndrome. If your pain is only in the butt, this could be a tight piriformis. If you cannot get into this position, this is due to tight muscles that may lead to this condition. **Repeat on the other side. If at any time the pain is too severe to attempt this test, call your doctor for evaluation.**

If these are your symptoms	You may suffer from	Do this test to confirm
Sensation on the inside of the knee that is painful to the touch, often accompanied by swelling.	Medial Meniscus Injury (Knee Pain)	Sit cross-legged yoga-style. If this causes pain on the inside of the knee, this could be a medial meniscus strain or tear, or tight, sore muscles that could be a precursor to the condition. If you cannot get into this position, this is due to tight muscles that may lead to this condition. **For severe, acute pain of the knee, first seek evaluation by your physician.**
Sensation of pain in the heel or the bottom of the foot.	Plantar Fasciitis (Heel Spur)	If the pain in the heel or bottom of the foot is worse in the morning and improves throughout the day, or if the pain is worse when you are walking without shoes, this could be plantar fasciitis or tight, sore muscles that could be a precursor to the condition.
Sensation of chronic, widespread pain with tenderness to light touch, often accompanied by fatigue. You may also feel tingling of the skin that feels like needles, as well as nerve pain and brain fog.	Fibromyalgia	Pain must be on both the left and right side of the body and both above and below the waist. This may also be tight, sore muscles or dehydration.

CHAPTER 3

overview of integrated positional therapy (IPT) wellness plans

In the following chapters you will find definitions of each of the thirteen conditions mentioned in this book. This will help you understand the mechanics of the condition that is causing your pain. Remember that all of these conditions are caused by certain muscles being too long and tight and some being too short and tight. These tight muscles pull the bones out of alignment, which can cause muscle pain, disc problems, nerve compressions, and tendonitis. For example, the headaches that I experienced as a result of my car accident were primarily due to muscle imbalances in the neck and shoulders. Once they were corrected, my headaches lessened and eventually went away.

You will also find a list of common causes for each of these conditions. In order for the body to feel better, it is important not only to reduce or eliminate the pain but also to eliminate the cause. This process often involves doing your daily activities in a slightly different way that stops the pain from returning. The old saying: "If you do what you always did, you get what you always got" applies here.

In my thirty-plus years of helping people, I have identified three activities that almost everybody does and which cause 50–60% of all the pain I treat. These activities are sitting in a chair, sitting in a car, and sitting at a computer. It is not the computer or the chair or the car causing the pain, but the way you are using those instruments. If you just do these three things a little bit more ergonomically, half of your pain can be eliminated. In the following pages I will show you how easy it is to obtain good results and how beneficial they can be.

Most people have the same or similar muscular imbalances in their bodies with some variations. This coincidence is explained by the fact that we do similar activities all day long. For example, most of us drive a car, sit at a computer, or slump in our chairs for a good part of the day. These positions will bring about similar muscular imbalances that will produce similar aches and pains. Almost everyone has tight neck and shoulder muscles whether they hurt or not. Neck and shoulder tightness is primarily caused by slumping over the computer or steering wheel or by walking with your head forward of the body. These positions all cause the neck and shoulders to be tight.

Almost everyone also has a pelvis that is out of balance, i.e. crooked. I have observed, in my thirty-plus years of treating pain, that if I bring the pelvis back into balance, the discs, the joints, the muscles, and other structures will also come back into balance and function normally, which will reduce or eliminate the pain in many other areas of the body as well.

Three primary pelvic imbalances lie at the root of many painful conditions in the body. These are an elevated pelvis, a rotated pelvis, and a tilted pelvis. Most people present with at least one of these, although most people present with all three in varying degrees. Let's take a closer look.

elevated pelvis

An elevated pelvis means that one hip is higher than the other. I have measured the elevated hip on my clients to be off anywhere from 1/8 of an inch to almost 2.5 inches. Typically, the higher the hip, the more painful the condition. People with an elevated pelvis will often be diagnosed as having one leg shorter than the other. This diagnosis is not usually correct. They have a functionally short leg but not a truly short leg. Although the leg is not truly shorter, it is functionally shorter when walking, which puts undue strain on the body structure. A functionally short leg means this is a temporary and correctable condition. I have only seen a few truly short legs in my practice. Most of these were from a broken leg that did not heal correctly, leaving the bones at different lengths.

Many people with an elevated pelvis and thus a functionally short leg will be told to get a heel lift to help even out the hip. Sometimes this strategy works, but oftentimes it does not. This strategy merely treats the symptom and not the cause. So what can cause an elevated pelvis? Muscle imbalances are the culprit. The two main muscles involved in this condition are the quadratus lumborum and the psoas. Either of these muscles, when they become short due to overuse or prolonged sitting, can elevate the pelvis, causing a functionally short leg. An elevated pelvis not only contributes to low back pain but to hip, knee, and foot pain as well.

rotated pelvis

A rotation in the pelvis can be either inward or outward. Typically when one side goes inward, the other side goes outward. These rotations can be anywhere to slight or quite pronounced. If you lie down on your back and either one or both of your legs and feet turn out, that can be an indication of a rotated pelvis.

The muscle imbalances that can cause a rotated pelvis are the hip abductor group of muscles on the outside of the upper leg and the external rotator group of muscles that are located deep in the butt tissue. When these muscles become short, they may rotate the pelvis. These groups of muscles not only contribute to low back pain but sciatica, hip, groin, and knee pain.

tilted pelvis

A tilted pelvis can be either forward or backward. A forward tilt is called an anterior pelvic tilt, and a backward tilt is called a posterior pelvic tilt. The most common is the forward tilt. The tilt can be anywhere from slight to pronounced.

The muscle imbalances that cause a forward tilt are the psoas—a deep muscle in the middle of the body—and the rectus femoris, which is one of the quadricep muscles in the upper leg. These are also called the hip flexor muscles.

The muscle imbalances that can cause a posterior tilt are the gluteal muscle group in the butt and the hamstrings on the back of the upper leg.

In either case, these imbalances will cause an exaggerated lumbar curve and compress the structures in the low back, putting undue strain on the entire body structure. In my opinion, a tilted pelvis is the primary cause of low back pain in many people.

Most people will have at least one of these imbalances, and many have all three. I will teach you four stretches that, when practiced consistently, usually bring the pelvis back into balance.

The treatment protocols listed for each condition evolved over thirty years to ensure safe, effective, easy application and were designed to fit your busy schedule. They only take minutes a day and will give you the tools to effectively deal with your muscular pains. Some of these protocols are about prevention, and some are proactive in reducing or eliminating the pain in your body. Doing each one consistently and gently is important. None of these stretches should hurt.

You will notice that many of the protocols are similar. Most include the four hip stretches to balance the pelvis. Whether you have a pain in the foot or the head, the root cause is often an unbalanced pelvis.

I want to take some time here to further discuss slackening a muscle. Most of us are familiar with stretching a muscle, but nobody thinks about slackening a muscle. A good analogy would be to think of a string. If I take the two ends of a string and pull them farther apart, this is called stretching. Slackening a muscle is taking the two ends of the string and bringing them closer together. This brings the muscle into slack. Where slack is present, tension is not. When our muscles are not tense, we will not feel pain. This position of slack must be held for two minutes or more in order for the muscle memory to take effect and keep the muscle loose. This often feels like a miracle, as the pain simply seems to disappear.

Remember the exercise in chapter 1 where we looked for a tender spot in the shoulder? That was a demonstration of putting a muscle in slack.

You can try this for yourself to feel what it is like to have a muscle in slack.

Take your left hand and gently place it on your right shoulder. Find a seam on your shirt that runs toward your neck. Somewhere along that seam, press into the tissue with a finger on your left hand. You will probably feel that it is sore, bumpy, or tight. This indicates a muscle imbalance in the region. Now keep your left hand where it is but stop pressing the tissue. Take your right arm and gently rest the forearm on top of your head. Completely relax it in that position. Hold it there for two minutes, which lets the muscle “reset” itself.

With your left hand, press the tissue again. It should feel softer and less painful. If it still hurts, move the arm into slightly different positions until the tissue feels better. You just put that muscle into slack.

These protocols are designed to treat the whole body and not only the site of the pain. By treating the whole body and removing the root cause, Integrated Positional Therapy obtains longer-lasting results.

how soon can I expect results?

In many cases of pain caused by muscle imbalances, short-term relief is immediate. Rebalancing the muscles usually gives a muscle 80–100% relief almost immediately, and the effects are cumulative. **The more you do it, the better the results.**

You can achieve long-term relief in three to five months if you are diligent with your exercises. That is how long it typically takes to retrain muscles—not a lot of time considering how long it took you to acquire these imbalances. **Performing the exercises consistently brings the best results.**

If the muscle imbalances have been present a long time, sometimes inflammation is as well. The Wellness Plans will rebalance the muscles and, in time, reduce or clear up the inflammation.

Lack of water can also be a factor in muscular pain. Many people do not drink enough water to adequately hydrate their cells. Muscles that do not get enough water ache more than muscles that are well hydrated. Also, the discs need to be well hydrated to maintain their softness and avoid pinching or irritating a nerve. Good disc health is dependent on adequate water intake.

Remember that caffeine and alcohol are diuretics, which means they take water out of the body. It is fine to have these things in moderation, but remember to drink even more water. People will overlook the basics like drinking water, and it is often the cause of many aches and pains. In general, drink half your body weight in ounces every day. Adequate fluid intake will help reduce the frequency of your pain and lead to better overall health. It can take up to six weeks to rehydrate, so please be patient. See chapter 17 for information on adequate water intake.

You will achieve superior benefits by performing the stretches correctly.

how to stretch for maximum benefit

Humans are the only species that stretch into pain! Stretching should feel good. If you watch a cat or a dog stretch, you will see that they experience no strain and that they look happy and relaxed. When you watch people stretch, you will often notice that they look strained and are working hard. What is the difference between animals and people when it comes to stretching? Animals listen to their bodies. People listen to their brains. The human brain keeps telling us if a little stretch feels good, a bigger stretch is even better. This mistake will often lead to pain.

My observations as a therapist have shown that bringing muscles back into balance requires only consistent, moderate stretches that feel good. **If you have soreness the next day, or if the stretch you are performing is painful, you have probably overstretched your muscles.** This is especially so if you have stretched a muscle that was already too long.

Stretching a muscle too deeply can lead to:

- Muscle tears
- Strained tendons and sprained ligaments
- Muscle weakness
- Joint dysfunction
- Inflammation

To achieve the most benefit from your stretching program, follow these guidelines:

- **Warm up the muscles before stretching.** This means you have to make the muscles warmer by raising the body temperature at least one degree. This warm-up should include some type of aerobic activity. Muscles stretch better when they are warm.
- **Stretch muscles to 75% or less of your maximum effort.** Muscles respond better to a stretch in the midrange than at their end range. Do not overstretch or stretch into pain.
- **Hold each stretch for 30–60 seconds,** but make sure you are not straining. Holding the stretch longer will stretch both the muscle and the other soft tissue surrounding the muscle. If you cannot hold the stretch for a minute, you might be stretching too deeply.
- **Do not bounce in a stretch.** This can lead to muscle tears.
- **Modify a stretch if necessary.** I will show you some modifications in this book. The stretches and modifications are all in the back of the book in the appendices. Do not hesitate to make further modifications. Remember that your stretching should feel good.

Caution: Never stretch into a painful position. You will achieve better results by being gentle. The goal is not to stretch as far as possible but to slightly increase range of motion. Done every day, the results can be dramatic and permanent.

Finally, although the protocols in this manual are effective, sometimes medical attention is required. **If the protocols are not working or you are getting worse, stop doing the exercises and please see your health care provider.**

CHAPTER 4

IPT wellness plan for tension-type headaches and migraines

headache is one of the most common reasons people seek medical help. In the United States alone, we spend an estimated $50–70 billion on headaches every year. That figure includes medical visits, alternative therapies, and over-the-counter pain medication.

Recent research shows that most headaches are probably a combination of tension and migraine. Whether the headache is caused by the muscle tension or the muscle tension results from the headache, treating that muscle tension can provide significant relief from the pain.

Tension-type headaches are often due to muscle imbalances in the neck and shoulder muscles. This means the tight muscles are either too long or too short and pull or compress other structures in this area, leading to pain. Even though a person experiences the pain in the head, the cause is often in the neck or shoulder area.

Many migraine headaches are also aggravated by muscle imbalances, but some are not. Other factors for migraine are diet, brain chemical imbalances, and hormonal imbalances. This chapter addresses migraines and headaches caused by muscle imbalances. *If the protocols listed in this book are not working, check with your health care provider, as you might have a migraine not caused by muscle imbalances or dehydration.*

You can improve or eliminate your headaches with a little awareness and some self-care. It is vital to first identify and correct the common everyday activities that are the source of muscle strain in the neck and shoulders that can lead to a headache. Many things you do every day may lead to pain and spasm in the muscles of the head, neck, or shoulders.

Maintaining good posture is essential in correcting muscle imbalances that can lead to headaches.

Another major factor in the cause of headaches is dehydration. Many people do not drink enough water to adequately hydrate their cells. Muscles that do not get enough water ache more than muscles that are well hydrated. If you feel a headache coming on, immediately drink two large glasses of water. Prompt fluid intake will sometimes stop the headache. In general, drink half your body weight in ounces every day. This may help reduce the frequency of your headaches and lead to better overall health. Fully hydrating the body can take up to six weeks, so please be patient.

Stretching the neck muscles every day is also important. Many people have a head-forward posture, which will put quite a strain on the neck muscles. A tight neck can lead to a headache. Many people walk into my office rubbing their neck and saying that they hold all their stress in their neck. While this is true, it is not the kind of stress most people think about. It is not so much "I got a ticket," "the boss yelled at me," or "the car broke down." This kind of emotional stress can of course add to the tension and pain in the neck and head. The real source, however, is mostly a mechanical stress of having the head and/or arms forward of the body when either sitting or standing. Bad posture is responsible for a great amount of the stress and tightness in the neck that can lead to a headache.

Stretching the chest muscles every day and strengthening the upper back will start to train your head to come back over the shoulders. We are a head forward society because we spend a lot of time bent forward. Training your head to align with your shoulders may significantly reduce the amount of headaches you experience.

By adopting the Wellness Plan in this chapter, you can eliminate or significantly reduce the number and severity of your headaches. If after practicing the Wellness Plan you still have no improvement, see your health care provider for further assessment.

symptoms:

A tension headache is felt as pain, tightness, or pressure around the head. The pain is sometimes described as throbbing or aching and can affect the front, top, back, or side of the head. A person feels the pain in the neck, upper back, eyes, jaw, or other muscle groups in the body. It may also radiate from other areas like the shoulders or upper back.

common causes:

Many lifestyle habits can contribute to a headache. The following are some of the most common I have come across in my practice.

- **Poor posture,** especially head forward of the body or arms held extended for long periods of time. These postures are typical of driving and computer positions. They put a lot of strain on the neck and shoulder muscles that can lead to a headache.
- **Emotional or mental stress, anxiety, TMJ, and/or teeth grinding at night.** This kind of stress makes your tight muscles even tighter. Try the breathing exercise described in chapter 17.
- **Fatigue and/or lack of sleep.** Fatigue upsets the chemical balance in the body and can lead to a headache. Try to get seven to eight hours of uninterrupted sleep.

- **Dehydration.** Lack of water can make your joints and/or muscles ache a lot more. See chapter 17 for instructions for proper hydration.
- **Eyestrain.** Eyestrain can cause a headache due to muscle imbalances around the eyes. If you wear glasses, make sure your prescription is up to date; if you do not wear glasses, see your eye doctor, as you might need them. Periodically give your eyes a rest. While at the computer, take a break and stare out the window for a few minutes. This shift in attention gives the eyes a different focal point and helps to relieve eyestrain.
- **Caffeine withdrawal.** When giving up caffeine, always do so slowly. Slowly coming off caffeine and keeping well hydrated can mitigate the effects of withdrawal.
- **Hunger.** Low blood sugar can also lead to a headache. Eat a balanced diet at regular intervals to keep the blood sugar even. Do not skip meals. Protein helps to keep blood sugar levels more even.
- **Reading in bed with head propped up.** This is a common practice that leads to many headaches. This position strains the neck and shoulder muscles and adversely affects the discs in the cervical spine.

With a little awareness and by following the Wellness Plan in this book, you can easily make the changes in your life that may help stop your headaches from returning.

conventional medical approach

Standard medical treatments for headaches often include painkillers, muscle relaxants, and antidepressants. Remember that these drugs do not cure headaches; rather, they alleviate the symptoms for a while. They do not address two of the biggest factors of headaches—dehydration and muscle imbalances.

IPT wellness plan for tension-type headaches and migraines

MUSCLE REBALANCING: This section explains the exercises you need to practice to correct the muscle imbalances that are causing your pain. By doing these exercises now and continuing to do them as instructed, you will make your short muscles longer and your long muscles shorter, bringing them back into balance.

four stretches to balance the pelvis (appendix b)

These stretches will help to bring the body structure back into balance, thus eliminating a major cause of aches and pains. They're designed to stretch the muscles or muscle groups that are typically too short in most people and pull the pelvis out of alignment. A crooked pelvis affects all the areas of the body and is often a major cause of neck strain and thus headaches, as many headaches are caused by tight neck muscles. Do these stretches three times a day and hold them for a minute each.

three neck stretches (appendix c)

These stretches will loosen the muscles in the neck and shoulders and allow more blood and oxygen to flow to the head and neck. Stretching these muscles takes only a few minutes and is a great habit to cultivate, as you will feel less pain and stiffness in the neck and will be more alert. Consistent practice will reduce or eliminate the cause of many headaches. Gently stretch the neck muscles three times a day.

slacken the jaw (appendix d)

Slackening the jaw will help to loosen the masseter muscle in the jaw, which is usually quite tight and short in most people. This tight muscle can refer pain to the head and/or pull the jaw out of alignment, which can then lead to a headache. Do this five times a day until the symptoms subside.

slacken the shoulders (levator scapula & upper trapezius; appendix e)

Slackening the shoulders will relieve tension in the shoulders, especially the upper trap and levator scapula muscle. These areas are tight and sore in most people. Do this exercise anytime you feel tension in your shoulders or neck and at least five times a day. Do not do this exercise if it hurts to put your arm on top of your head.

shoulder shrugs (appendix e)

Shoulder shrugs will help relax your shoulder and neck muscles and bring more blood and oxygen to the area, reducing tension and pain. This will also help you feel more alert. Repeat several times throughout the day.

strengthen rhomboids and latissimus dorsi (appendix e)

Strengthening the rhomboids and the lats will help to shorten and strengthen the muscles between the shoulder blades and the muscles below the shoulder blades, thus training the muscles to bring the head over the shoulders, improving the posture and reducing the strain on the neck. Do this three to five times a day. Hold for one minute.

stretch the chest (pectoralis major & minor; appendix f)

In most people the chest muscles are too short and the rhomboids between the shoulder blades are too long, which gives a person a head-forward, bent-over look with rounded shoulders. Stretching the chest muscles will release tension between the shoulder blades and open up the chest, which will make a person stand up straighter. When a person stands straight, the bones in the cervical spine hold up the head, and the neck muscles can then relax. Hold for at least one to two minutes. Do this exercise three times a day.

slacken the chest (appendix f)

Slackening the chest muscles will relax the muscles in the chest, especially the pectoralis minor muscle. Relaxing these muscles helps people with shoulders rounded forward to bring them back into better alignment and will help bring the head over the shoulders, thus reducing strain on the neck. Totally relax and hold that position for two minutes. Do this twice a day.

SUPPORTIVE LIFESTYLE: This part of your Wellness Plan is designed to address the root of the problem and to relieve habitual muscle imbalances to avoid aggravating the condition as you go about your daily life.

check sitting, driving, and computer positions (appendix a)

Correcting your posture while sitting, driving, and working at a computer will ensure the pelvis stays in balance, your head is aligned over your shoulders, and that you are not causing more stress on the neck, shoulders, and lower and upper back. These common activities are responsible for a great amount of the pain in your life. These activities will often make your body crooked and lead to muscle imbalances that could lead to a headache and possible lumbar or cervical disc problems. By slightly changing the way you perform these activities, you will keep the body in alignment. This will help ensure that once the pain is relieved, it does not come back.

walk or stand holding your wrist behind your back

This stance will ensure that you have good posture when you are standing or walking. It will bring the head over the shoulders, open the chest, and correct a forward pelvic tilt. Use this position when you are walking slowly or standing in one place. When walking briskly, swing your arms naturally to help move and clean out your lymphatic system, which is the body's sewer system.

keep elbows close to the body when performing daily activities

Holding the arms away from the body for long periods can lead to tight, sore muscles in many areas of your body and cause a headache. In addition to your driving and computer positions, other common activities that cause muscle strain are using the phone, and household activities like chopping vegetables or vacuuming. Performing your daily activities with your elbows close by your side will eliminate or prevent a lot of your pain.

stay well hydrated

One of the most common causes of headache is dehydration. Even slight dehydration can cause a headache. If the headache is just starting, immediately drink two large glasses of water. This will often help. If you already have a headache, start hydrating as soon as possible. See chapter 17 for instructions on how to drink water and how much. Rehydrating the body can take up to six weeks.

keep the neck as warm as possible

Wearing a collar, turtleneck shirt, or scarf around your neck, even inside the house, can be helpful. Keeping the neck as warm as possible will help keep the neck muscles loose and reduce pain. A cold breeze on the neck is a factor in many headaches and stiff necks.

regular exercise

Light, regular exercise such as walking every day for at least twenty minutes can help with your headache by increasing your circulation. Exercise also releases certain neurotransmitters (chemicals) in the brain that can help reduce or eliminate pain.

heat the shoulders and neck for twenty minutes

Use a heating pad on the neck and shoulders every day for about twenty minutes. Applying warmth will help to relax the muscles in the area and bring more blood and oxygen to the tissues. Continue until the symptoms subside.

success story

A thirty-seven-year-old woman came to me for help with her headaches. She had suffered from these headaches once a week for a period of five years. On a pain scale of 1–10, her headaches were a 7 or 8. She was following her doctor's advice and treating them with over-the-counter pain medications. She did not have a headache the day I saw her. They occurred mostly on the right side of her head in the temple, forehead, and behind the eye. Headaches in this area almost always originate in the upper trap muscles, which are on the top of the shoulder. I needed to find out what she was doing to make this muscle so tight that it produced a headache.

The upper trap muscle gets tight with any head-forward posture, typically driving or sitting at a computer incorrectly. Sure enough, she had a desk job. I asked her to describe her workstation setup. She showed me how she sat at her computer. Her head was far forward while looking at her screen, which was too low, and her arm was extended too far away from her body when holding the mouse. The entire posture put tremendous strain on the upper trap muscle. The muscle was sore to the touch, which is an indication that it was tight and likely causing the headaches. I put her in the "slacken the shoulder" position (see Appendix E), and immediately the sore spot in her upper trap muscle felt about 90% better. I held it there for two minutes. When I took her out of that position and touched the spot on her shoulder, the pain was 100% gone. She exclaimed that it felt like a miracle had just happened. "No miracle," I said. "Just good science."

Another big factor with headaches is a lack of water. Even a 1% decline in normal hydration levels could trigger a headache.

I asked her if she was well hydrated, and she said, "Yes, as a matter of fact I am drinking all day long."

"Good," I said. "What are you drinking?"

"I drink between six and eight cups of coffee a day."

She didn't realize that coffee is a diuretic that actually takes water out of the body and dehydrates it. Caffeine also makes your muscles tighter and can give you a headache if you consume too much. I explained to her that the tight muscles in her shoulder and the lack of water in the tissues were more than likely the main causes of her headaches. I explained that because rehydrating the tissues can take four to six weeks, cutting back on the coffee to no more than two cups a day was imperative. I also told her to start drinking a lot of water. Avoiding coffee altogether would be even better in this case.

I put her on the Wellness Plan described above. I explained that this protocol usually works well but that she would have to be consistent. Since pain is the great motivator, I was confident she would follow my instructions.

I saw her again three months after that appointment. She reported that her headaches were mostly gone, occurring only now and then and usually when she had too much coffee. She also reported the side effects of feeling happier and having better memory recall.

This Wellness Plan has worked for many hundreds of my clients who suffer from headaches.

CHAPTER 5

IPT wellness plan for temporomandibular joint disorder (TMJ)

TMJ is the common abbreviation for temporomandibular joint disorder. This joint allows you to open and close your mouth, chew, and speak. An improperly functioning joint can be very painful. Muscle imbalances in the neck, face, and jaw muscles often start with a crooked pelvis because the spine sits on the pelvis. If the pelvis is crooked, the spine is crooked. This means the tight muscles are either too long or too short and pull or compress other structures in this area, leading to pain.

The temporomandibular joint, sometimes called the "jaw joint," is in front of the ear. The joint attaches the lower jaw to the skull. If you place two fingers on your jaw in front of the ear and chew, you can feel the joint moving. TMJ is a condition where tight muscles put pressure on the joint, and in more severe cases even pull it out of joint.

An estimated ten million Americans suffer from this condition. You can have tight, sore jaw muscles and not have TMJ. The protocol for treating a tight jaw is the same as for TMJ. A tight jaw is often a precursor to TMJ. You can improve or eliminate your TMJ or tight jaw with a little awareness and some self-care. But first you must identify and correct the common everyday activities that are causing muscle strain in the neck and shoulders that can lead to TMJ. Many activities you do every day may lead to pain and spasm either in the muscles of the jaw or those of the head, neck, or shoulders.

The strain of slumping, which pushes your head forward of your body, can lead to TMJ.

Stretching the neck muscles every day is also important. Many people have a head-forward posture, which will put quite a strain on the neck. A tight neck can lead to TMJ. Bad posture is responsible for a great amount of the stress in the neck.

By adopting the Wellness Plan in this chapter, you can eliminate or significantly reduce your TMJ pain. If after practicing the Wellness Plan you still have no improvement, see your health care provider for further assessment.

symptoms:

TMJ is felt as pain in the jaw joint and/or the surrounding area. It may also be felt as ear pain and/or ringing in the ears. When the joint moves, you may hear sounds, such as clicking and/or popping. Other symptoms include swelling of the face or mouth, headache, and dizziness. Your bite may feel uncomfortable. The jaw may also become locked in either the open or closed position.

common causes:

Many lifestyle habits can contribute to TMJ. The following are some of the most common I have come across in my practice:

- Tight muscles around the jaw (especially the masseter), grinding teeth, and stress. Even emotional stress can cause tight muscles. This kind of stress, in fact, makes your tight muscles even tighter. Try the breathing exercise described in chapter 17.
- Chewing gum, poor posture, reading in bed, cradling a phone between your ear and shoulder, or playing a wind or string instrument. These activities put a lot of strain on the neck, shoulder, and jaw muscles that can lead to TMJ. (See Wellness Plan.)

With a little awareness and by following the Wellness Plan in this book, you can easily make the changes in your life that will help alleviate your TMJ symptoms.

conventional medical approach

Standard medical treatments for TMJ often include painkillers, muscle relaxants, cortisone shots, or Botox injections. If these are not successful, surgery or corrective dental treatments are prescribed. Remember that the drugs and surgery do not always cure TMJ; rather, they alleviate the symptoms for a while. They do not address the primary cause of TMJ—muscle imbalances.

IPT wellness plan for temporomandibular joint disorder (tmj)

MUSCLE REBALANCING: This section provides the exercises to practice to correct the muscle imbalances that are causing your pain. By doing these exercises now and continuing to do them as instructed, you will make your short muscles longer and your long muscles shorter, bringing them back into balance.

four stretches to balance the pelvis (appendix b)

These stretches will help to bring the body structure back into balance, thus eliminating a major cause of aches and pains. These exercises are designed to stretch the muscles or muscle groups that are typically too short in most people and pull the pelvis out of alignment. When the pelvis is crooked, it affects all the areas of the body. A pelvis that is out of alignment is often a cause of TMJ and headaches. Do these stretches three times a day. Hold for one minute each.

three neck stretches (appendix c)

These stretches will loosen the muscles in the neck and shoulders and allow more blood and oxygen to flow to the head and neck. Doing these stretches takes only a few minutes and is a great habit to cultivate, as you will feel less pain and stiffness in the neck and will be more alert. Consistent practice will reduce or eliminate a major cause of TMJ. Gently stretch the neck muscles three times a day.

slacken the jaw (appendix d)

Slackening the jaw will help to loosen the masseter muscle in the jaw, which is usually very tight and short in most people. This tight muscle can refer pain to the head and/or pull the jaw out of alignment, which can then lead to TMJ. Do this five times a day until the symptoms subside. Hold for two minutes. Do not perform this exercise if it worsens the pain.

slacken the shoulders (levator scapula & upper trapezius; appendix e)

Slackening the shoulders will relieve tension in the shoulders, especially the upper traps and levator scapula muscles. These tight muscles can contribute to TMJ. These areas are tight and sore in most people. Do this exercise anytime you feel tension in your shoulders or neck and at least five times a day. Hold for two minutes. Do not do this exercise if it hurts to put your arm on top of your head.

shoulder shrugs (appendix e)

Shoulder shrugs will help relax your shoulder and neck muscles and bring more blood and oxygen to the area, which will reduce tension and pain. This will also help you feel more alert. Repeat several times throughout the day.

strengthen rhomboids and latissimus dorsi (appendix e)

Strengthening the rhomboids and the lats will help to shorten and strengthen the muscles between the shoulder blades and the muscles below the shoulder blades, thus training the muscles to bring the head over the shoulders, improving the posture and reducing the strain on the neck and jaw. Hold for at least one minute. Do this three to five times a day.

stretch the chest (pectoralis major & minor; appendix f)

In most people the chest muscles are too short and the rhomboids between the shoulder blades are too long, which give a person a head-forward, bent-over look with rounded shoulders. Stretching the chest muscles will release tension between the shoulder blades and open up the chest, which will make a person stand up straighter. When a person stands straight, the bones in the cervical spine hold up the head, and the neck and jaw muscles can relax. Hold for at least one to two minutes. Do this exercise twice a day.

slacken the chest (appendix f)

Slackening the chest muscles will relax the muscles in the chest, especially the pectoralis minor muscle. Relaxing these muscles helps people with shoulders rounded forward to bring them back into better alignment and will help to bring the head over the shoulders, thus reducing strain on the neck and jaw. Totally relax and hold that position for two minutes. Do this twice a day.

SUPPORTIVE LIFESTYLE: This part of your Wellness Plan is designed to address the root of the problem and to relieve habitual muscle imbalances to avoid aggravating the condition as you go about your daily life.

check sitting, driving, and computer positions (appendix a)

Correcting your posture while sitting, driving, and working at a computer will ensure the pelvis stays in balance and that you are not causing more stress on the neck, jaw, shoulders, and lower and upper back. These common activities are responsible for a great amount of the pain in your life. Doing these activities the incorrect way will make your body crooked and lead to muscle imbalances and possible lumbar or cervical disc problems. By slightly changing the way you perform these activities, you will keep the body in alignment and help ensure that once the pain is relieved it does not come back.

keep elbows close to the body when performing daily activities

Holding the arms away from the body for long periods can lead to tight, sore muscles in many areas of your body like the jaw, neck, and shoulders. In addition to your driving and computer positions, other common activities that cause muscle strain are using the phone, and household activities like chopping vegetables or vacuuming. Performing your daily activities with your elbows close by your side will eliminate or prevent a lot of your pain.

DO NOT CHEW GUM

Chewing gum can tighten the muscles in the jaw and worsen the condition.

slow, deep breathing for 10–15 minutes (see chapter 17)

Slow, deep breathing relaxes the nervous system and thus relaxes the muscles in the jaw. Done just before bedtime, this exercise will help to reduce grinding of the teeth at night, which is a major cause of TMJ. Do this at least twice a day.

success story

A forty-five-year-old male came to see me who had a stressful job and was suffering with jaw pain that was diagnosed as TMJ. He was using a bite plate that his dentist recommended, and his doctor had recommended surgery. His pain level was 5 on a scale of 10. He had been experiencing these symptoms for about a year. His pain was mostly in the jaw, which made a clicking noise when opening and closing.

When I touched the masseter muscle, which is the big muscle in the jaw area, he felt pain with only light pressure. I slackened the jaw and pressed the tissue again, and he said that he now felt no pain at all. It was gone. After holding that position for two minutes, he said that he felt much better.

I still wanted to know what was giving him these muscle imbalances in the jaw and causing the pain. The cause is usually poor computer or driving positions. When I asked him to describe his office setup, it appeared to be a pretty good ergonomic setup. Upon further inquiry, I found out that he liked to read in bed at night propped up against the headboard with his head far forward. This position can cause a lot of pain in the neck, face, or jaw.

I explained the Wellness Plan above to him and told him he needed to be consistent to get the results he wanted. His jaw pain went away almost immediately and he adopted the Wellness Plan, which kept the condition from coming back.

I have not only used this protocol to help many of my clients, but I also eliminated my own TMJ from many years of playing the trumpet.

CHAPTER 6

IPT wellness plan for cervical muscle strain (neck pain)

The neck or cervical spine is that part of the body that connects the head to the trunk. It is comprised of muscles, nerves, arteries, bones, and discs. These discs act like shock absorbers between the cervical vertebrae.

Neck pain can occur due to muscular tightness in both the neck and upper back or as a result of compressed nerves in this region. Almost everyone will experience a tight, sore neck in his or her lifetime. In my thirty-plus years of experience, I have only worked with a handful of people who did not have a tight neck.

Pain felt in the neck is usually caused by muscle imbalances in the neck, shoulder, or upper back. This means the tight muscles are either too long or too short and pull or compress other structures in this area, leading to the pain. A crooked pelvis is a contributor to neck pain because the spine sits on the pelvis.

You can improve or eliminate your neck pain with a little awareness and some self-care. Identifying and correcting the common everyday activities causing muscle strain in the neck, shoulders, or upper back are vital. Many activities you do every day may lead to pain and spasm in the muscles of the neck, shoulders, or upper back.

A good place to start avoiding neck pain is by practicing good posture. Note how you sit at work, in front of a computer, and when driving. Maintaining proper posture will allow your spinal column to do the work of holding up your head rather than your neck muscles.

Lack of water can also be a factor in neck pain. The discs need to be well hydrated to maintain their softness and avoid pinching or irritating a nerve. Good disc health is dependent on adequate water intake.

It is also very important to stretch the neck muscles every day. Many people have a head-forward posture, which will put quite a strain on the neck. Bad posture is responsible for a great amount of the stress in the neck.

By adopting the Wellness Plan in this chapter, you can eliminate or significantly reduce your neck pain. If after practicing the Wellness Plan you still have no improvement, see your health care provider for further assessment.

symptoms:

Pain in the neck could be described as an ache, tightness, burning, or stabbing. This condition can be acute or chronic. It is often better or worse in certain positions such as lying down, sitting, or standing. It can also radiate to other parts of the body such as down the arms or the upper back or head.

common causes:

Many lifestyle habits can contribute to neck pain. The following are some of the most common I have come across in my practice:

- Improper sitting positions, driving positions, standing positions, and computer positions lead to head-forward posture that can cause cervical muscle strain and perhaps lead to a disc issue.
- Emotional stress can also aggravate cervical muscle strain. Try the breathing exercise described in chapter 17.
- Reading in bed.

With a little awareness and by following the Wellness Plan in this book, you can easily make the changes in your life that will help to alleviate your symptoms of neck pain.

conventional medical approach

Standard medical treatments for neck pain often include painkillers and muscle relaxants. Surgery is sometimes prescribed for nerve compression or herniated discs. Remember that the drugs and surgery do not always cure neck pain; rather, they alleviate symptoms for a while. They do not address the primary cause of neck pain—muscle imbalances.

IPT wellness plan for cervical muscle strain (neck pain)

MUSCLE REBALANCING: This section provides the exercises you need to practice to correct the muscle imbalances that are causing your pain. By doing these exercises now, and continuing to do them as instructed, you will make your short muscles longer and your long muscles shorter, bringing them back into balance.

four stretches to balance the pelvis (appendix b)

These stretches will help to bring the body structure back into balance, thus eliminating a major cause of aches and pains. These exercises are designed to stretch the muscles or muscle groups that are typically too short in most people and pull the pelvis out of alignment. A crooked pelvis affects all the areas of the body. A pelvis that is out of alignment is often a major cause of neck strain and thus headaches, as many headaches are caused by tight neck muscles. Do these stretches three times a day. Hold for one minute each.

three neck stretches (appendix c)

These stretches will loosen the muscles in the neck and shoulders and allow more blood and oxygen to flow to the head and neck. It only takes a few minutes to do these stretches, and doing them is a great habit to cultivate, as you will feel less pain and stiffness in the neck and will be more alert. Consistent practice will reduce or eliminate the cause of a great amount of your neck pain. Gently stretch the neck muscles three times a day.

slacken the shoulders (levator scapula & upper trapezius; appendix e)

Slackening the shoulders will relieve tension in the shoulders and neck, especially the upper traps and levator scapula. These areas are tight and sore in most people. Do this exercise anytime you feel any tension in your shoulders or neck and at least five times a day. Hold for two minutes. Do not do this exercise if it hurts to put your arm on top of your head.

shoulder shrugs (appendix e)

Shoulder shrugs will help relax your shoulder and neck muscles and bring more blood and oxygen to the area, reducing tension and pain. This will also help you feel more alert. Repeat several times throughout the day.

strengthen rhomboids and latissimus dorsi (appendix e)

Strengthening the rhomboids and lats will help to shorten and strengthen the muscles between the shoulder blades, as well as the muscles below the blades, thus training the muscles to bring the head over the shoulders, improving posture and reducing strain on the neck. Hold for one minute. Do this three times a day.

stretch the chest (pectoralis major & minor; appendix f)

In most people the chest muscles are too short and the rhomboids between the shoulder blades are too long, which give a person a head-forward, bent-over look with rounded shoulders. Stretching the chest muscles will release tension between the shoulder blades and open up the chest, which will make a person stand up straighter. When a person stands straight, the bones in the cervical spine hold up the head and the neck muscles can relax. Hold for at least one to two minutes. Do this exercise twice a day.

slacken the chest (appendix f)

Slackening the chest muscles will relax the muscles in the chest, especially the pectoralis minor muscle. Relaxing these muscles helps people with shoulders rounded forward to bring them back into better alignment and will help to bring the head over the shoulders, thus reducing strain on the neck. Totally relax and hold that position for two minutes. Do this twice a day.

SUPPORTIVE LIFESTYLE: This part of your Wellness Plan is designed to address the root of the problem and to relieve habitual muscle imbalances to avoid aggravating the condition as you go about your daily life.

check sitting, driving, and computer positions (appendix a)

Correcting your posture while sitting, driving, and working at a computer will ensure the pelvis stays in balance and that you are not causing more stress on the neck, shoulders, and lower and upper back. These common activities are responsible for a great amount of the pain in your life. Doing these activities the incorrect way will make your body crooked and lead to muscle imbalances and possible lumbar or cervical disc problems. By slightly changing the way you perform these activities, you will keep the body in alignment and help ensure that once the pain is relieved, it does not come back.

walk or stand holding your wrist behind your back

This stance will ensure that you have good posture when you are standing or walking. It will bring the head over the shoulders, which will reduce or prevent neck pain. This will also open the chest and start to unround your shoulders. This position should be used when you are walking slowly or standing in one place. When walking briskly, swing your arms naturally, which helps to move and clean out your lymphatic system, the body's sewer system.

keep elbows close to the body when performing daily activities

Holding the arms away from the body for long periods can lead to tight, sore muscles in many areas of your body like the neck. In addition to your driving and computer positions, other common activities that cause muscle strain are using the phone, and household activities like chopping vegetables or vacuuming. Performing your daily activities with your elbows close by your side will help to eliminate or prevent a lot of your pain.

keep the neck as warm as possible

Wear a collar, turtleneck shirt, or scarf around your neck, even inside the house. Keeping the neck as warm as possible will help keep the neck muscles loose and reduce pain. A cold breeze on the neck is a factor in many headaches and stiff necks.

heat the shoulders and neck for twenty minutes

Use a heating pad on the neck and shoulders every day for about twenty minutes. Applying warmth will help to relax the muscles in the area and bring more blood and oxygen to the tissues. Continue until the symptoms subside.

keep well hydrated

Dehydration is a factor in cervical neck strain. Even slight dehydration can cause the neck muscles to ache. Many people are dehydrated. See chapter 17 for instructions on how to drink water and how much. Rehydrating the body can take up to six weeks.

regular exercise

Light, regular exercise, such as walking every day for at least twenty minutes, can help with your neck pain by increasing your circulation. Exercise also releases certain neurotransmitters in the brain that can help eliminate pain.

success story

A woman in her fifties came to me complaining of pain in her neck, which she had suffered with for twenty years following a car accident. She had initially been diagnosed with whiplash. The pain was in the back of the neck on the left side and was a 6 on a scale of 10, bad enough to often wake her at night. She had seen specialists all over the country and in Europe. Despite their best efforts, her pain remained.

I had her point to exactly where she felt the pain. I performed the "slacken the shoulder" move and then gently did the three neck stretches. When I asked her how her neck felt after that, she looked surprised. She admitted that she didn't think I would to be able to help her, but the pain in her neck was gone. She was even a bit angry. She said, "You mean I suffered for twenty years and this is all somebody needed to do?" She was sure that her pain was going to come back, so I explained the Wellness Plan to her and the importance of being diligent. I also explained how whiplash and the resulting pain is all about muscle imbalances. Once you know which muscles are too long and tight and which muscles are short and tight, reducing or eliminating pain becomes quite easy.

Almost every client I see has at least a tight neck, if not a painful one. The above Wellness Plan takes only a few minutes a day and is a great practice for everyone to adopt.

CHAPTER 7

IPT wellness plan for thoracic outlet syndrome (TOS)

The thoracic outlet is the space between the collarbone and the first rib. Thoracic outlet syndrome (TOS) is a compression of the nerves and/or blood vessels that affects the brachial plexus (nerves that pass into the arms from the neck) and various nerves and blood vessels in that space. This compression is due to muscle imbalances in the neck, chest, back, and pelvis when not due to the presence of an extra rib called a cervical rib. As a result, the tight muscles are either too long or too short and pull or compress other structures in this area, which leads to the pain in the arms or hand.

You can improve or eliminate TOS with a little awareness and some self-care. It is vital to first identify and correct the common everyday activities that are causing muscle strain in the neck and shoulders that can lead to TOS. Many activities you do every day may lead to pain and spasm in the muscles of the head, neck, shoulders, and back.

Maintaining excellent posture is a key first step in relieving the strain on muscles causing TOS. By correcting your computer and driving positions, you will bring your head over your shoulders, giving yourself good posture. Your bones (the spinal column) will be holding up your head, which will help take the strain off the muscles. Holding your arms on the steering wheel at the ten o'clock and two o'clock positions strains the muscles that cause TOS. Instead, bring your arms down to the four o'clock and eight o'clock positions to take the strain off the muscles responsible for causing TOS.

Stretching the neck muscles every day is vital. This is especially true of the muscles on the side of the neck (scalenes). These muscles attach on the first rib. When tight, they pull up that rib, decreasing the space in the thoracic outlet and possibly causing a compression of the nerves and blood vessels, which can result in pain and tingling down the arm.

Many people have a head-forward posture that causes quite a strain on the neck. A tight neck can lead to pain, fatigue, discomfort, and possibly TOS. Bad posture is responsible for a great amount of the muscular tension in the neck.

It is also important to stretch and slacken the chest muscles. A tight, short pectoralis minor muscle in the chest can bring on numbness and tingling down the arm.

By adopting the Wellness Plan in this chapter, you can eliminate or significantly reduce your TOS. If after practicing the Wellness Plan you still have no improvement, see your health care provider for further assessment.

symptoms:

Thoracic outlet syndrome is a sensation of pain, numbness, tingling, weakness, burning, or coldness in the arm and/or hand caused by pressure on the nerves and/or blood vessels in the thoracic outlet. It can occur on one side of the body or both. The pain can be in the whole hand or just part of the hand, as in only the fourth and fifth fingers.

Tingling, pain, or numbness indicates a compression of the nerves. Coldness indicates a compression of the blood vessels.

The symptoms of TOS are often confused with carpal tunnel, as they can be similar. By performing the tests in chapter 2, you will likely be able to tell which condition you have. Some people will have both TOS and carpal tunnel at the same time.

common causes:

Many lifestyle habits can contribute to thoracic outlet syndrome. The following are some of the most common I have come across in my practice:

- Repetitive activities that require the arms to be held over the head or outstretched
- Poor posture, especially head forward
- Improper computer and driving positions
- Cradling phone between shoulder and ear or holding phone to ear
- Riding a bike
- Whiplash
- Gardening

These activities can all cause muscle imbalances in the neck, shoulders, and pelvis, which can cause compression of the brachial plexus in the thoracic outlet.

With a little awareness and by following the Wellness Plan in this book, you can easily make the changes in your life that will help alleviate the symptoms of TOS.

conventional medical approach

Standard medical treatments for thoracic outlet syndrome often include painkillers and muscle relaxants. Physical therapy is also widely prescribed for this condition. Surgery is sometimes prescribed for nerve compression or blood vessel constriction. Remember that drugs and surgery do not cure thoracic outlet syndrome unless it is caused by the extra rib, called a "cervical rib." Rather, drugs and surgery alleviate the symptoms for a while. They do not address the primary cause of TOS—muscle imbalances.

IPT wellness plan for thoracic outlet syndrome (TOS)

MUSCLE REBALANCING: This section provides the exercises you need to practice to correct the muscle imbalances causing your pain. By doing these exercises now, and continuing to do them as instructed, you will make your short muscles longer and your long muscles shorter, bringing them back into balance.

four stretches to balance the pelvis (appendix b)

These stretches will help to bring the body structure back into balance, thus eliminating a major cause of aches and pains. These exercises are designed to stretch the muscles or muscle groups that are typically too short in most people and pull the pelvis out of alignment. A crooked pelvis affects all the areas of the body. A pelvis that is out of alignment is often a major cause of neck strain that can lead to thoracic outlet syndrome. Do these stretches three times a day. Hold for one minute each.

three neck stretches (appendix c)

These stretches will loosen the muscles in the neck and shoulders and allow more blood and oxygen to flow to the head and brain, reducing pain in the neck and head. Stretching the scalenes, the muscles on the side of the neck, is especially important to relieve the pain from TOS. Stretching the scalenes creates more space in the thoracic outlet, taking pressure off the nerves. Gently stretch the neck muscles three times a day.

slacken the shoulders (levator scapula & upper trapezius; appendix e)

Slackening the shoulders will relieve tension in the shoulders, especially the upper traps and levator scapula. These areas are tight and sore in most people. Do this exercise anytime you feel tension in your shoulders or neck and at least five times a day. Hold for two minutes. Do not do this exercise if it hurts to put your arm on top of your head. This move might bring on some tingling, which is okay for short periods of time.

shoulder shrugs (appendix e)

Shoulder shrugs will help relax your shoulder and neck muscles and bring more blood and oxygen to the area, which will help reduce tension and pain. This will also help you feel more alert. This exercise will create more space in your thoracic outlet and take pressure off the nerves causing the symptoms. Repeat several times throughout the day.

strengthen rhomboids and latissimus dorsi (appendix e)

Strengthening the rhomboids and lats will help to shorten and strengthen the muscles between the shoulder blades and the muscles below the shoulder blades, thus training the muscles to bring the head over the shoulders, improving your posture, reducing strain on your neck, and creating more space in the thoracic outlet. Do this three times a day. Hold for one minute.

stretch the chest (pectoralis major & minor; appendix f)

In most people the chest muscles are too short and the rhomboids between the shoulder blades are too long, which give a person a head-forward, bent-over look with rounded shoulders. Stretching the chest muscles will release tension between the shoulder blades and open up the chest, which will make a person stand up straighter. When a person stands up straight, the bones in the cervical spine hold up the head and the neck muscles can relax, allowing more space in the thoracic outlet. Hold for at least one to two minutes. Do this exercise twice a day.

slacken the chest (appendix f)

Slackening the chest muscles will relax the muscles in the chest, especially the pectoralis minor muscle. Relaxing these muscles helps people with shoulders rounded forward to bring them back into better alignment and will help to bring the head over the shoulders, thus reducing strain on the neck and taking strain off the nerves in the thoracic outlet. Totally relax and hold that position for two minutes. Do this exercise twice a day.

SUPPORTIVE LIFESTYLE: This part of your Wellness Plan is designed to address the root of the problem and to relieve habitual muscle imbalances to avoid aggravating the condition as you go about your daily life.

check sitting, driving, and computer positions (appendix a)

Correcting your posture while sitting, driving, and working at a computer will ensure the pelvis stays in balance and that you are not causing more stress on the neck, shoulders, and lower and upper back that can lead to TOS. These common activities are responsible for a great amount of the pain in your life. Doing these activities incorrectly will make your body crooked and lead to muscle imbalances and possible lumbar or cervical disc problems. By slightly changing the way you perform these activities, you will keep the body in alignment and help alleviate the symptoms associated with TOS.

walk or stand holding your wrist behind your back

This stance will ensure that you have good posture when you are standing or walking. It will bring the head over the shoulders, open the chest, and correct any pelvic tilt. This position should be used when you are walking slowly or standing in one place. Do not perform this exercise if your symptoms of TOS worsen while doing it. When walking briskly, swing your arms naturally, which will help to move and clean out your lymphatic system, the body's sewer system.

keep elbows close to the body when performing daily activities

Holding the arms away from the body for long periods can lead to tight, sore muscles in many areas of your body. In addition to your driving and computer positions, other common activities that cause muscle strain are using the phone, and household activities like chopping vegetables or vacuuming. Performing your daily activities with your elbows close by your side will eliminate or prevent a lot of the symptoms of TOS.

heat your shoulders and thoracic outlet area

Put a heating pad on your shoulders and upper chest for twenty minutes. Do this every day until your symptoms subside.

success story

A woman in her twenties came to me suffering from numbness and tingling in her right hand and arm. She had been diagnosed with thoracic outlet syndrome and had experienced these symptoms for six months. Although she was not in much pain, the numbness and tingling made it difficult for her to do her work as a massage therapist.

First, I wanted to make sure that she really did have TOS, as carpal tunnel symptoms are similar. I had her raise both hands over her head and wiggle her fingers. This is the test for TOS. Sure enough, in about twenty seconds, she started to have numbness and tingling.

The thoracic outlet is the space between the first rib and the collarbone. Symptoms develop when there is not enough space. The first thing I did was to see if her pelvis was crooked. I found that it was elevated about 1.5 inches. Since the spine sits on the pelvis, her spine was also crooked. Since the ribs attach to the spine, her ribs became crooked, reducing the space in the thoracic outlet.

I did the four stretches to balance the pelvis, the three neck stretches, and the slacken the chest move. I had her repeat the test for TOS by raising her hands over her head. She had no tingling this time.

The movements I did on her corrected her muscle imbalances and opened up the space in the thoracic outlet, preventing further nerve compression. I further made sure that she was sitting correctly, as described in Appendix A.

I explained the Wellness Plan listed above and told her it was very important to practice this every day so that her symptoms did not return.

CHAPTER 8

IPT wellness plan for thoracic muscle strain (upper back pain)

Upper back pain is a common condition that affects millions of people. The pain radiates anywhere from just below the neck to all the way down to the bottom rib. The most common area is right between the shoulder blades. The spine is often divided into three sections. The cervical spine, which consists of seven vertebrae, is in the neck; the lumbar spine, consisting of five vertebrae, is in the low back region; and the thoracic spine, which consists of twelve vertebrae, makes up the upper and middle back.

Pain in the upper back is usually caused by muscle imbalances in the neck, shoulder, upper back, and chest. This means the tight muscles are either too long or too short and pull or compress other structures in this area, causing pain. A crooked pelvis is a contributor to upper back pain because the spine sits on the pelvis and thus becomes crooked as well.

If a nerve in this area is compressed due to muscle imbalances or injury, that pain may radiate and be felt in the arms or chest.

Many activities a person does every day can lead to pain in the muscles of the head, neck, shoulders, or back. Learning to have and maintain excellent posture is an ideal place to start.

Lack of water can also be a factor in upper back pain. The discs need to be well hydrated to maintain their softness and avoid pinching or irritating a nerve. Discs should be about 80% water. Good disc health is dependent on adequate water. Interestingly, a recent study found that 70% of herniated discs cause no pain in the body.

By adopting the Wellness Plan in this chapter, you can eliminate or significantly reduce your upper back pain. If after practicing the Wellness Plan you still have no improvement, see your health care provider for further assessment.

symptoms:

Pain in the upper back is often described as an ache, tightness, burning, or stabbing. This condition can be acute or chronic. It is often better in certain positions such as lying down or standing or sitting. It is usually worse with long periods of sitting in a chair or reading in bed. The pain may also radiate down the arms.

common causes:

Many lifestyle habits can contribute to upper back pain. Improper sitting positions, driving positions, and computer positions lead to head forward posture that can cause thoracic muscle strain and perhaps lead to a disc issue. Muscle imbalances in the upper back (thoracic region) can lead to pain and tightness, especially between the shoulder blades.

The following conditions are caused by muscle imbalances and are a major source of upper back pain:

- Unbalanced pelvis
- Tight, short pectoral muscles
- Overstretched, strained rhomboids
- Forward-rotated shoulders
- Head-forward posture
- Some disc problems

With a little awareness and by following the Wellness Plan in this book, you can easily make the changes in your life that will help alleviate your upper back pain.

conventional medical approach

Standard medical treatments for upper back pain often include painkillers and muscle relaxants. Physical therapy is often prescribed. Surgery is sometimes prescribed for nerve compression or herniated discs. Remember that the drugs and surgery do not always cure upper back pain; rather, they alleviate the symptoms for a while. They do not address one of the biggest factors of upper back pain—muscle imbalances.

IPT wellness plan for thoracic muscle strain (upper back pain)

MUSCLE REBALANCING: This section provides the exercises you need to practice to correct the muscle imbalances that are causing your pain. By doing these exercises now and continuing to do them as instructed, you will make your short muscles longer and your long muscles shorter, bringing them back into balance.

four stretches to balance the pelvis (appendix b)

These stretches will help to bring the body structure back into balance, thus eliminating a major cause of aches and pains. These exercises are designed to stretch the muscles or muscle groups that are typically too short in most people and which pull the pelvis out of alignment. When the pelvis is crooked, all areas of the body are affected. A pelvis that is out of alignment is often a major cause of neck strain and upper back pain because those muscles are out of balance. Do these stretches three times a day. Hold for a minute each.

three neck stretches (appendix c)

These stretches will loosen the muscles in the neck, shoulders, and upper back to allow more blood and oxygen to flow to the head and neck. Take a few minutes to do these stretches, making them a habit, as you will feel less pain and stiffness in the neck and will be more alert. Consistent practice will reduce or eliminate the cause of a great amount of your upper back pain. Gently stretch the neck muscles three times a day.

slacken the shoulders (levator scapula & upper trapezius; appendix e)

Slackening the shoulders will relieve tension in the shoulders and neck, especially the upper trap and levator scapula muscle. These areas are tight and sore in most people. Do this exercise anytime you feel any tension in your shoulders or neck and at least five times a day. Do not do this exercise if it hurts to put your arm on top of your head. Hold for two minutes.

shoulder shrugs (appendix e)

Shoulder shrugs will help relax your shoulder and neck muscles and bring more blood and oxygen to the area, which will reduce tension and pain. This will also help you feel more alert. Repeat several times throughout the day.

strengthen rhomboids and latissimus dorsi (appendix e)

Strengthening the rhomboids and the lats will help to shorten and strengthen the muscles between the shoulder blades and the muscles below the blades, thus training the muscles to bring the head over the shoulders, improving posture and "reducing strain on the upper back. Do this three times a day for one minute.

stretch the chest (pectoralis major & minor; appendix f)

In most people the chest muscles are too short and the rhomboids between the shoulder blades are too long, which give a person a head-forward, bent-over look with rounded shoulders. Stretching the chest muscles will release tension between the shoulder blades and open up the chest, which will make a person stand up straighter. When a person stands straight, the bones in the cervical spine hold up the head and the upper back muscles can relax. Hold for at least two minutes. Do this exercise three to five times a day.

SUPPORTIVE LIFESTYLE: This part of your Wellness Plan is designed to address the root of the problem and to relieve habitual muscle imbalances to avoid aggravating the condition as you go about your daily life.

check sitting, driving, and computer positions (appendix a)

Correcting your posture while sitting, driving, and working at a computer will ensure the pelvis stays in balance and that you are not causing more stress on the neck, shoulders, and lower and upper back. These common activities are responsible for a great amount of the pain in your life. Doing these activities the incorrect way will make your body crooked and lead to muscle imbalances and possible lumbar or cervical disc problems. By slightly changing the way you perform these activities, you will keep the body in alignment and help ensure that once the pain is relieved, it does not come back.

walk or stand holding your wrist behind your back

This stance will ensure that you have good posture when you are standing or walking. It will bring the head over the shoulders, which will reduce or prevent upper back pain. This will also open the chest. This position should be used when you are walking slowly or standing in one place. When walking briskly, swing your arms naturally, which will help to move and clean out your lymphatic system, the body's sewer system.

keep elbows close to the body when performing daily activities

Holding the arms away from the body for long periods can lead to tight, sore muscles in many areas of your body like the upper back. In addition to your driving and computer positions, other common activities that cause muscle strain are using the phone, and household activities like chopping vegetables or vacuuming. Performing your daily activities with your elbows close by your side will help eliminate or prevent a lot of your pain.

heat upper back for twenty minutes

Use a heating pad on the upper back every day for about twenty minutes. Applying warmth will help to relax the muscles in the area and bring more blood and oxygen to the tissues. Continue until the symptoms subside.

keep well hydrated

Dehydration is a factor in thoracic muscle strain. Even slight dehydration can cause the upper back muscles to ache. Many people are dehydrated. See chapter 17 for instructions on how much water to drink. Rehydrating can take up to six weeks.

regular exercise

Light, regular exercise such as walking every day for at least twenty minutes can help with your upper back pain by increasing your circulation. Exercise also releases certain neurotransmitters in the brain that can help eliminate pain.

success story

A man in his thirties came to see me complaining of a sharp pain between his shoulder blades. The pain was mostly on the right side. I asked him what he did for a living, as a person's job will often give me a clue as to how the person acquired the pain. He told me that he sat in front of a computer all day.

He had been experiencing this pain for about two years on and off, but lately it had been constant and sometimes would even wake him up at night. It seemed to be getting worse.

I asked him what he was doing to try and alleviate the pain. He said he had tried massage, which did give him some temporary relief. He said when the pain was extra bad, he would take a painkiller that would give him six hours of relief.

Pain between the shoulder blades is common and is almost always due to sitting in a slumped position with the shoulders rounded forward and reaching too far for the mouse and/or keyboard.

When a person sits slumped, their chest muscles become very short and the muscles between the shoulder blades long, overstretched, and tight. Try this for yourself. Round your shoulders forward and then touch the tissue between the shoulder blades. They will feel tight and painful.

When a muscle is too long, overstretched, and tight, massaging it will make it feel better but will not make it shorter and thus correct the root of the problem.

In order to make the tissue between the shoulder blades relax, this patient needed to stretch the short tissue of the chest muscles. When I did that, his pain was noticeably better. Sometimes when inflammation is involved, eliminating all the pain will take a little longer.

I also did four stretches to bring his pelvis back into balance and showed him how to do these stretches himself. Remember, a crooked pelvis gives you a crooked spine, which then leads to upper or low back pain.

I showed him the proper sitting, computer, and driving positions that would help keep his pelvis straight. I taught him to place his arms at the four o'clock and eight o'clock positions when driving and at the computer.

I stressed the importance of the Wellness Plan. He left my office with his pain about 80% reduced. In a follow-up appointment he stated that he had followed my advice, rearranging his computer setup and moving the steering wheel in his car to a different position. His pain had thus gone away. He did confess that sometimes he didn't practice the Wellness Plan and the pain started to creep back. But he felt confident, knowing he had the tools to keep the pain permanently at bay.

CHAPTER 9

IPT wellness plan for epicondylitis, lateral or medial (tennis or golfer's elbow)

Lateral epicondylitis is inflammation and pain at the site of the lateral epicondyle, where the wrist extensor muscles attach by way of a tendon to the little bony bump on the outside of the elbow. A tendon attaches the extensor muscles to the elbow. This condition is often called tennis elbow.

Medial epicondylitis is inflammation and pain at the site of the medial epicondyle, where the wrist flexor muscles attach by way of a tendon to the little bony bump on the inside of the elbow. This condition is often called golfer's elbow. Muscle imbalances in the forearm muscles mean the tight muscles are either too long or too short and pull or compress other structures in this area, which leads to the elbow pain.

You can improve or eliminate epicondylitis with a little awareness and some self-care. It is vital to first identify and correct the common everyday activities that are causing muscle strain in the forearms that can lead to epicondylitis. Many activities you do every day may lead to pain and spasm in the muscles of the forearms.

With tennis or golfer's elbow, the muscles and tendons that are involved are used in almost every daily activity—everything from brushing your teeth to typing at your computer, any activity that involves using your hands. Proper posture and ergonomics will certainly help, but these tendons are in constant use throughout the day. Learning to keep your wrist straight and unbent during all daily activities is crucially important. A bent wrist in either direction puts strain on the elbow tendons and aggravates epicondylitis. If you have trouble keeping your wrist straight, use a wrist brace, which can be bought at any pharmacy, to help keep the wrist straight until the symptoms subside.

Another important practice is to slacken these tendons every day by performing the stretch and slacken the forearms exercises as described in the Wellness Plan. This practice will take the strain off the tendon so it can begin to heal.

Lack of water can also be a factor in epicondylitis. Many people do not drink enough water to adequately hydrate their cells. Muscles that do not get enough water ache more than muscles that are well hydrated. Also, the elbow joint needs to be well hydrated to maintain good lubrication. Good joint health is dependent on adequate water.

Do not rest your arms on the armrest of a chair. Resting your arms on armrests can interfere with the motion of the forearm muscles as they contract and relax, aggravating epicondylitis.

Rest is still one of nature's best healing methods. Since tennis or golfer's elbow is usually an overuse injury, resting your arms and hands, or at least reducing the amount of activity, will speed up the healing process.

By adopting the Wellness Plan in this chapter, you can eliminate or significantly reduce the symptoms of epicondylitis. If after practicing the Wellness Plan you still have no improvement, see your health care provider for further assessment.

symptoms:

Epicondylitis presents as pain or stiffness at the site of the elbow, sometimes radiating to other parts of the arm. The pain is often worse when typing or squeezing objects. The pain usually occurs in the dominant arm, although it can be in the other arm or both arms.

common causes:

Many lifestyle habits can contribute to tennis or golfer's elbow. The following are some of the most common I have come across in my practice:

- Working at a computer
- Playing a musical instrument
- Knitting
- Cutting vegetables
- Carpentry
- Tennis
- Golf
- Painting
- Lifting heavy objects
- Gripping objects too firmly

These activities can all cause muscle imbalances in the forearm muscles that attach to the elbow. Limiting these activities when you have a sore elbow will speed up the recovery process.

With a little awareness and by following the Wellness Plan in this book, you can make the changes in your life that will help to alleviate the pain associated with epicondylitis.

conventional medical approach

Standard medical treatments for tennis or golfer's elbow often include painkillers, muscle relaxants, and anti-inflammatory drugs. Physical therapy is also widely prescribed for this condition. Surgery is sometimes prescribed to clean up damaged tissue. Remember that drugs and surgery do not always cure epicondylitis; rather, they alleviate the symptoms for a while. They do not address one of the biggest factors of epicondylitis—muscle imbalances.

IPT wellness plan for epicondylitis, lateral or medial (tennis or golfer's elbow)

MUSCLE REBALANCING: This section provides the exercises you need to practice to correct the muscle imbalances that are causing your pain. By doing these exercises now, and continuing to do them as instructed, you will make your short muscles longer and your long muscles shorter, bringing them back into balance.

slacken the thumb (hand squeeze; appendix g)

Slackening the thumb will release the muscle in the thumb called the pollicis and the other muscles on the palm side of the hand. Although it is not the primary muscle involved in epicondylitis, this muscle is usually tight and sore as well. Hold for two minutes. Do this as many times throughout the day as you can.

elbow tendon release (appendix g)

Releasing the elbow tendons will take strain off the muscles in the forearm that can contribute to epicondylitis. Hold for two minutes. Repeat three times a day.

slacken and stretch the forearm (wrist flexors and extensors; appendix g)

Slackening and stretching the forearm muscles will release the tight muscles that can contribute to epicondylitis. These tight muscles will pull on the elbow and may bring on symptoms. Hold each position for two minutes. Repeat ten times a day, reducing the number of repetitions as the pain subsides. If one of the directions causes pain, only do the one that feels good.

SUPPORTIVE LIFESTYLE: This part of your Wellness Plan is designed to address the root of the problem and to relieve habitual muscle imbalances to avoid aggravating the condition as you go about your daily life.

check sitting, driving, and computer positions (appendix a)

Correcting your posture while sitting, driving, and working at a computer will ensure the pelvis stays in balance and that you are not causing more stress on the neck, shoulders, and lower and upper back by holding your arms and hands in positions that can indirectly bring on the symptoms of epicondylitis. These common activities are responsible for a great amount of the pain in your life. Doing these activities the incorrect way will make your body crooked and lead to muscle imbalances and possible lumbar or cervical disc problems. By slightly changing the way you perform these activities, you will keep the body in alignment and help ensure that once the pain is relieved, it does not come back.

keep elbows close to the body when performing daily activities

Holding the arms away from the body for long periods can lead to tight, sore muscles in many areas of your body. In addition to your driving and computer positions, other common activities that cause muscle strain are using the phone, and household activities like chopping vegetables or vacuuming. Performing your daily activities with your elbows close by your side will eliminate or prevent a lot of your pain. Do not rest your arms on the armrests of a chair, as this can aggravate epicondylitis.

keep your wrists straight during all daily activities

For activities that you must do during the day, keep your wrists straight. A bent wrist puts pressure on the elbow tendons and will bring on symptoms. If you have difficulty keeping a straight wrist, use a wrist brace for this purpose. Try to be aware of your wrist position so that you don't become dependent on the brace. Use it as a short-term tool during recovery and to help you learn proper wrist position.

rest your arms

Activities involving your hands are the main cause of this condition. Limiting or avoiding using your hands for a while in conjunction with the other exercises listed here will help alleviate the pain.

heat forearms for twenty minutes

Use a heating pad on your forearms every day for twenty minutes. Continue until your symptoms subside.

ice your elbow

If you have significant pain in the elbow, icing it for ten minutes will often bring quick relief. You can ice your elbow at the same time as you heat the forearm.

success story

A man in his forties came to see me with a diagnosis from his doctor of tennis elbow (lateral epicondylitis). He had been suffering with this condition for about a year. His job involved sitting at a computer all day and he was also a tennis player. More people today get tennis elbow from their computer than they actually do from tennis. Both these activities can cause tennis elbow.

This condition is sometimes hard to clear up because we have to use the muscles in the forearm a lot in our daily activities, thus reinjuring the elbow every day.

The tissue at the site of the elbow was very sore to the touch. I performed the move to slacken and stretch the forearm. I touched the tissue again, and the man's pain was gone for the first time in a year.

I explained to him that although the pain was gone, the inflammation was still there and he could easily reinjure those muscles. I advised him to give up tennis for four weeks and showed him how to slacken the forearm muscles. I had him do this slackening ten times a day for two minutes each time for a period of two weeks. Then he was to reduce the frequency to five times a day for maintenance.

When I saw him two months later, he reported that as long as he did the Wellness Plan, his pain did not return. If he stopped following the plan, the pain would start to creep back.

As a massage therapist, I use my hands a lot and it would be easy to get tennis elbow. I slacken my forearms five times a day to keep myself pain-free.

CHAPTER 10

IPT wellness plan for carpal tunnel syndrome (CTS)

The carpal tunnel is a small space located on the palm side of the wrist. It is formed on the bottom by the wrist bones and on the top by the retinaculum, which is a band of connective tissue. The median nerve and several tendons that help bend your fingers run through this space, like going through a tunnel. Carpal tunnel syndrome (CTS) is a condition in which the median nerve is compressed at the wrist in the tunnel. Bending the wrist decreases the size of the tunnel. The median nerve is the only nerve that runs through the tunnel. The pain associated with CTS is often due to muscle imbalances in the forearm muscles unless brought on by pregnancy. The tight muscles in the forearm are either too long or too short and pull or compress other structures in this area, especially the median nerve, which leads to the pain or numbness.

You can improve or eliminate CTS with a little awareness and some self-care. It is vital to first identify and correct the common everyday activities that cause muscle strain in the arms and hands that can lead to CTS.

The muscles and tendons involved in carpal tunnel syndrome are ones used in almost every daily activity—everything from brushing your teeth to typing at your computer. CTS is aggravated by any activity that involves using your hands. Proper posture and ergonomics will certainly help, but these tendons and muscles are in constant use throughout the day. Keeping your wrist straight and unbent during all daily activities is vitally important. A bent wrist in either direction puts strain on the median nerve, aggravating CTS. If you have trouble keeping your wrist straight, use a wrist brace, which can be bought at any pharmacy, to help keep the wrist from bending until the symptoms subside. It is especially important to wear the wrist brace at night, as many people sleep with a bent wrist, which can bring on the symptoms.

Slackening the area of the carpal tunnel is important to do every day. This will often take the strain off the median nerve so it can begin to heal. In the beginning, you should do this ten times a day. You can decrease that number as your symptoms subside.

Also have your health care provider check your vitamin B-12 levels. Low levels of B-12 are sometimes associated with carpal tunnel syndrome.

Lack of water can also be a factor in CTS. Many people do not drink enough water to adequately hydrate their cells. Muscles that do not get enough water ache more than muscles that are well hydrated. Also, the joints need to be well hydrated to maintain their lubrication. Good joint health is dependent on adequate water intake.

Do not rest your arms on the armrest of a chair. Resting your arms on armrests can interfere with the motion of the forearm muscles and tendons as they contract and relax. This position can aggravate carpal tunnel syndrome.

Rest is still one of nature's best healing methods. Since CTS is usually an overuse injury, resting your arms and hands, or at least reducing the amount of activity, will speed up the healing process.

Soaking the area in Epsom salts and warm water will often bring relief.

By adopting the Wellness Plan in this chapter, you can eliminate or significantly reduce CTS. If after practicing the Wellness Plan you still have no improvement, see your health care provider for further assessment.

symptoms:

Carpal tunnel syndrome is a sensation of pain, numbness, tingling, burning, or weakness in the hand and fingers caused by pressure on the median nerve in the carpal tunnel. This condition especially affects the thumb and the first two fingers. It is often accompanied by loss of grip strength, making it hard to hold a cup or a phone, and can include swelling of the hand.

common causes:

Many lifestyle habits can contribute to carpal tunnel syndrome. The following are some of the most common I have come across in my practice:

- Sitting at a computer
- Playing a musical instrument
- Knitting
- Cutting vegetables
- Carpentry
- Sleeping with bent wrists
- Painting
- Lifting heavy objects
- Gripping objects too firmly
- Biking

These activities can all cause muscle imbalances in the forearm muscles, affecting the carpal tunnel. Limiting these activities when you have carpal tunnel syndrome will speed up the recovery process

conventional medical approach

Standard medical treatments for carpal tunnel syndrome often include painkillers, muscle relaxants, and anti-inflammatory drugs. Physical therapy is also widely prescribed for this condition. Surgery is sometimes prescribed to take the pressure off the median nerve, which causes the pain and numbness. Remember that drugs and surgery do not always cure CTS; rather, they alleviate the symptoms for a while. They do not address the biggest cause of CTS—muscle imbalances.

IPT wellness plan for carpal tunnel syndrome (CTS)

MUSCLE REBALANCING: This section provides the exercises you need to practice to correct the muscle imbalances that are causing your pain. By doing these exercises now, and continuing to do them as instructed, you will make your short muscles longer and your long muscles shorter, bringing them back into balance.

slacken the thumb (hand squeeze; appendix g)

Slackening the thumb will release the muscle in the thumb called the pollicis and the other muscles on the palm side of the hand. This will also create more space in the carpal tunnel, taking pressure off the median nerve. Hold for two minutes. Do this exercise as many times throughout the day as you can.

slacken and stretch the forearm (wrist flexors and extensors; appendix g)

Slackening and stretching the forearm muscles will release the tight forearm muscles that can contribute to CTS. Tight forearm muscles may decrease the space in the carpal tunnel and bring on symptoms. Hold each position for two minutes. Do this ten times a day, reducing the number of repetitions as the pain subsides. If one of the directions causes pain, only do the one that feels good.

SUPPORTIVE LIFESTYLE: This part of your Wellness Plan is designed to address the root of the problem and to relieve habitual muscle imbalances to avoid aggravating the condition as you go about your daily life.

check sitting, driving, and computer positions (appendix a)

Correcting your posture while sitting, driving, and working at a computer will ensure the pelvis stays in balance and that you are not causing more stress on the neck, shoulders, and lower and upper back that can indirectly lead to carpal tunnel syndrome by holding your arms and hands in positions that can bring on the symptoms. By slightly changing the way you perform these activities, you will keep the body in alignment and help ensure that once the pain is relieved, it does not come back.

rest arms and hands

Cut back on the daily activities that require the use of your hands as much as possible until your symptoms are improved. Typing, knitting, playing an instrument, and chopping vegetables are typical activities that make your forearm muscles tight and bring on symptoms. Rest is still nature's great healer.

keep your wrists straight during all daily activities

For activities that you must do during the day, keep your wrists straight. A bent wrist puts pressure on the median nerve and will bring on symptoms. If you have difficulty keeping a straight wrist, use a wrist brace for this purpose. Try to be aware of your wrist position so that you don't become dependent on the brace. Use it as a short-term tool during recovery and to help you learn proper wrist position.

wear a wrist brace at night to keep your wrist straight

Carpal tunnel is often worse at night because most people sleep with bent wrists. This position will put pressure on the median nerve all night. Wearing a wrist brace at night will help.

heat forearm and hands

Use a heating pad on your hands, wrists, and forearms. Do this once or twice a day for at least twenty minutes. Continue until your symptoms subside.

check vitamin b-12 levels

Have your health care provider check your B-12 levels. Low levels of B-12 may be associated with carpal tunnel syndrome.

soak hands and wrists in epsom salts

Soak your hands and wrists in a little tub of warm water for twenty minutes a night for five nights. Make the water deep enough to cover your wrists. Use about one pound of Epsom salts to three to five gallons of water. Epsom salt is magnesium sulfate. It is a natural muscle relaxant and a natural anti-inflammatory.

success story

A woman in her twenties came to see me with a diagnosis of carpal tunnel syndrome. She had these symptoms for six months, and her doctor had recommended surgery. She worked at a desk job at the computer all day. Upon further inquiry, I found out she was also a knitter. Both of these activities can lead to carpal tunnel syndrome.

CTS is often hard to clear up, as the muscles involved are used often in our everyday life. I recommended she give up knitting for at least a month and that she wear a wrist brace to keep her wrist straight. A bent wrist will keep aggravating the median nerve. I told her to wear it while sleeping and during the day.

I showed her how to slacken the thumb, which will often relieve the symptoms of CTS. When I tried to slacken the forearm muscles, both directions were painful, so we did not pursue that exercise.

I told her to heat her forearm muscles every night for twenty minutes.

I also explained the importance of drinking enough water to keep the hand and wrist well lubricated.

She later reported to me that the symptoms of her carpal tunnel started to get a little better within four days and have continued to improve. At the time I spoke with her, she was hopeful that she would not need the surgery.

CHAPTER 11

IPT wellness plan for hip pain (bursitis)

The pain from this condition may be on the outer side of the upper leg and hip or the inside of the upper leg and hip, which is called the groin.

The hip joint attaches the leg to the torso. This is a ball and socket joint and allows for smooth movement when walking, if all is well. The pain may be caused by the joint itself or one of the structures around the joint such as the bursa, the tendons, the labrum, or the muscles surrounding the joint.

The front of the hip is commonly called the groin. This is the area where the inner thigh on the upper leg and the abdomen meet. This typically involves the hip adductors, hip flexors, and hip abductors. Pain often occurs when the muscles in the groin are stretched beyond their limits. Groin pain often indicates a problem with the hip joint.

Hip and groin pain are common in both athletes and yoga practitioners and are often due to muscular imbalances in the pelvis, legs, and low back. This means that the muscles in these areas are either too long or too short and pull or compress other structures in this area, leading to the pain.

You can improve or eliminate hip or groin pain with a little awareness and some self-care. It is vital to first identify and correct the common everyday activities that are causing muscle strain in the hip and groin that can lead to the pain. Many things you do every day may lead to pain and spasm in the muscles of the hip and groin.

One of the most common causes of these muscle imbalances is overusing certain muscles, which then makes them too short and tight. People who are active usually have tight, short hip flexors and abductors, and tight but too long adductors. This common muscle imbalance pattern pulls the pelvis out of alignment and can lead to hip and groin pain.

Many people walk and sit with their feet turned out. This puts a lot of strain on the hip and groin. It is important to correct the muscle imbalances that lead to people walking this way. Training the feet to go back to the neutral position, pointing straight ahead, is vital. Sitting with your toes turned in will help to correct muscles imbalances in the hip and groin that are causing your legs and feet to be rotated out. Do not stand or walk with your toes turned in. Just sit that way. Remember this should not hurt. If it does, you are turning in your feet too far.

Feet that turn out indicate the muscles on the outside of the leg are too short. Practicing the hip abductor stretch will lengthen those muscles and start to bring the feet straighter, taking the strain out of the hip and groin.

Lack of water can also be a factor in hip and groin pain. Many people do not drink enough water to adequately hydrate their cells. Muscles that do not get enough water ache more than muscles that are well hydrated. The hip joint needs to be well hydrated in order to keep it lubricated. That will reduce or eliminate any inflammation in the hip and/or groin. Good joint health is dependent on adequate water.

By adapting the Wellness Plan in this chapter you can eliminate or significantly reduce your hip or groin pain. If after practicing the Wellness Plan you still have no improvement, see your health care provider for further assessment.

symptoms:

Symptoms can be pain on the outside of the hip or in the groin area. Sometimes this pain is referred to this area from the low back. The pain can range from mild to severe, from sharp to a little achy. The pain may make walking difficult and is often worse with activity.

common causes:

Many lifestyle habits can contribute to hip or groin pain. The following are some of the most common I have come across in my practice:

- Sports Injuries
- Dancing
- Driving
- Yoga
- Weightlifting

These activities can all cause muscle imbalances in the hip or groin, which can lead to pain in this area. Limiting these activities when you have hip or groin pain will speed up the recovery process.

These conditions caused by muscle imbalances are a major source of hip or groin pain:

- Imbalanced pelvis
- External rotators too short
- Short abductors
- Long adductors

These physiological changes can also cause hip or groin pain:

- Hernia
- Bursitis
- Arthritis

conventional medical approach

Standard medical treatments for hip or groin pain often include painkillers, muscle relaxers, antidepressants, cortisone, and anti-inflammatories. Physical therapy is also widely prescribed for this condition. Surgery is sometimes prescribed if these measures are not working. Remember that the drugs or surgery don't always cure hip or groin pain; rather, they alleviate the symptoms for a while. They do not address the primary cause of the problem—muscle imbalances.

IPT wellness plan for hip pain (bursitis)

MUSCLE REBALANCING: This section provides the exercises you need to practice in order to correct the muscle imbalances that are causing your pain. By doing these exercises now and continuing to do them as instructed, you will make your short muscles longer and your long muscles shorter, bringing them back into balance.

four stretches to balance the pelvis (appendix b)

These stretches will help to bring the body structure back into balance, thus eliminating a major cause of aches and pains. They are designed to stretch the muscles or muscles groups that are typically too short in most people and pull the pelvis out of alignment. A crooked pelvis affects all the areas of the body. A pelvis that is out of alignment is often a major cause of hip or groin pain. Do these stretches three times a day. Hold for a minute each.

slacken the hip flexors (psoas & quadriceps; appendix h)

Lying on your back on the floor, bend at the hip 90 degrees and at the knees 90 degrees, resting the lower legs on a chair or sofa.

strengthen the hip extensors (hamstrings and gluteus maximus; appendix h)

The main hip extensor muscles are the hamstrings and gluteus maximus. These muscles are typically too weak in many people. Weak hip extensor muscles are a major cause of low back or hip pain. Do this strengthening exercise three or more times a day for at least one minute or longer. Don't practice this exercise if it causes pain.

strengthen the inside thighs (adductors; appendix i)

Sitting in a chair, fold a bed pillow in half and place it between the knees. Gently squeeze the knees together for five seconds. Repeat ten times, rest for a minute, and do ten more. Continue in this manner until you can do five sets of ten reps. This will strengthen the muscles on the inside of the upper leg.

SUPPORTIVE LIFESTYLE: This part of your Wellness Plan is designed to address the root of the problem and to relieve habitual muscle imbalances to avoid aggravating the condition as you go about your daily life.

check sitting, driving, and computer positions (appendix a)

Adjusting your sitting positions will ensure the hip stays in balance and that you are not causing more stress in the groin. Sitting is responsible for a great amount of the pain in your life. Sitting, driving, and typing on a computer the incorrect way will make your body crooked. By slightly changing the way you perform these activities, you will keep the body in alignment and help make sure once the pain is relieved, it does not come back. When driving, make sure your foot is straight on the gas pedal and not turned outward.

slacken the inside thighs (adductors; appendix i)

Most people sit with their legs and feet turned out to the sides. Sitting with your legs and feet slightly turned in will take strain off the hip and groin. Do not walk or stand like this. Do this only when sitting. Remember, this should not hurt. If it does, you are turning in your feet too far.

use heat on the thigh

Heat the hip and groin twenty minutes every night. These are the muscles on the outside of the upper leg (hip) and the inside of the upper leg (groin).

success story

A man in his thirties, a soccer player, came to me complaining of severe pain deep in the groin area on the right side. He said he'd had twinges of the pain for four months, but now it was debilitating. The pain was much worse when he was playing soccer and not so bad when he was sitting. He had seen his doctor, who ruled out a hernia and a labral tear.

I observed that the man's pelvis was quite out of balance. It was elevated and quite rotated. These conditions can cause a lot of strain in the hip and groin area. When I palpated the tissue on the inside of the leg, it felt ropy and tight, much like an overstretched rubber band.

I balanced the pelvis as much as I could and told him he would need to do some stretching at home so he could help resolve the rest of problem. I gave him the four stretches to balance the pelvis. I emphasized that he should do only these stretches until the pain subsided.

In addition to the tight muscles in the groin area, which were overstretched, he had some inflammation in the area. I told him that would probably clear up in a few weeks if he would follow the Wellness Plan and drink plenty of water.

His pain gradually subsided and he was able to play soccer again. It took about three months for him to recover. I emphasized that he should keep doing the Wellness Plan I gave him so he could continue to play soccer pain-free.

CHAPTER 12

IPT wellness plan for lumbar muscle strain (low back pain)

The lower back is a large area that connects the upper body to the lower body. Pain felt in the lower back is usually caused by muscle imbalances in this lumbar region. The tight muscles are either too long or too short and pull or compress other structures in this area, leading to the pain. Tight muscles will often pull the pelvis out of alignment and/or cause the spine to be crooked and/or cause a disc issue. Pain may also radiate from other areas like the mid or upper back.

Low back pain is very common. Almost everyone will experience low back pain at some time in their life. According to the *Journal of the American Osteopathic Association,* we spend $100 billion each year on this condition. Headache and low back pain are two of the most common reasons people seek medical attention.

You can improve or eliminate low back pain with a little awareness and some self-care. It is vital to first identify and correct the common everyday activities that cause the muscle strain that can lead to low back pain. Many activities you do every day may lead to pain in the muscles of the head, neck, shoulders, or back.

One of the most common causes of these muscle imbalances is simply poor posture and/or improper ergonomics. Slumping at your desk or in your car pushes your head forward of your body and rounds out the lower back, putting a lot of strain on your neck, shoulders, and low back, which will likely pull the pelvis out of alignment. Keeping your back rounded for long periods of time in your chair is a major factor in low back pain. I believe that half the back pain in the country would be eliminated if everyone sat with the proper support. By correcting your computer and driving positions, you will bring your head over your shoulders and straighten out your back, giving yourself good posture. Your bones (the spinal column) will be doing their job, which will help take the strain off the muscles.

Pelvic misalignment is common and often causes low back pain. The pelvis tends to be misaligned in three common ways: 1) it is higher on one side; 2) it is rotated; 3) it is tilted either forward or backward. Most people have at least one of these imbalances, and many have all three. The stretches described in the Wellness Plan for Lumbar Muscle Strain will help realign the pelvis.

Lack of water can also be a factor in low back pain. Many people do not drink enough water to adequately hydrate their cells. Muscles that do not get enough water ache more than muscles that are well hydrated. Also, the discs need to be well hydrated to maintain their softness and avoid pinching or irritating a nerve. Discs should be about 80% water. Good disc health is dependent on adequate water intake.

By adopting the Wellness Plan in this chapter, you can eliminate or significantly reduce your low back pain. If after practicing the Wellness Plan you still have no improvement, see your health care provider for further assessment.

symptoms:

Lumbar pain is pain in the low back that could be described as an ache, tightness, burning, or stabbing. This condition can be acute or chronic. It is often better in certain positions, such as lying down or standing or sitting. It may be painful to get up out of a chair or bed. The pain may also radiate down the legs and is often accompanied by pain in the groin.

common causes:

Many lifestyle habits can contribute to low back pain. The following are some of the most common I have come across in my practice:

- Long periods of improper standing
- Long periods of improper sitting
- Sports—especially one-sided sports like tennis and golf
- Lifting heavy objects

These activities can all cause muscle imbalances in the low back (lumbar region), which can lead to low back pain. Limiting these activities when you have lumbar muscle strain will speed up the recovery process.

The following conditions are caused by muscle imbalances and are a major source of low back pain:

- Unbalanced pelvis
- Tight, short quadriceps
- Externally rotated legs
- Some disc issues
- Stenosis

conventional medical approach

Standard medical treatments for low back pain often include painkillers, muscle relaxants, antidepressants, cortisone, and anti-inflammatory drugs. Physical therapy is also widely prescribed for this condition. Surgery is sometimes prescribed if other measures are not working. Remember that drugs and surgery do not cure low back pain; rather, they alleviate the symptoms for a while. They do not address the biggest cause of lumbar muscle strain—muscle imbalances.

IPT wellness plan for lumbar muscle strain (low back pain)

MUSCLE REBALANCING: This section provides the exercises you need to practice to correct the muscle imbalances causing your pain. By doing these exercises now and continuing to do them as instructed, you will make your short muscles longer and your long muscles shorter, bringing them back into balance.

four stretches to balance the pelvis (appendix b)

These stretches will help to bring the body structure back into balance, thus eliminating a major cause of aches and pains. These exercises are designed to stretch the muscles or muscle groups that are typically too short in most people and pull the pelvis out of alignment. When the pelvis is crooked, all areas of the body are affected. A pelvis that is out of alignment is often a major cause of neck strain and low back pain because those muscles are out of balance. Do these stretches three times a day. Hold for one minute each.

slacken the hip flexors (psoas and quadriceps; appendix h)

The hip flexor muscles are typically too short in most people. The very act of sitting in a chair, which we have done our entire lives, makes the hip flexors short. These short hip flexors will pull the pelvis forward, resulting in an anterior pelvic tilt, which can cause an exaggerated curve in the low back, low back pain, or disc problems. Slackening the hip flexors relaxes these muscles and lets the pelvis release back to neutral, which can alleviate pain. Do this slackening three or more times a day for at least two minutes or longer.

strengthen the hip extensors (hamstrings and gluteus maximus; appendix h)

The main hip extensor muscles are the hamstrings and gluteus maximus. These muscles are typically too weak in many people. Weak hip extensor muscles are a major cause of low back or hip pain. Do this strengthening exercise three or more times a day for at least one minute or longer. Don't practice this exercise if it causes pain.

half-frog (slacken the piriformis; appendix h)

The half-frog position will slacken the piriformis muscle and take strain off the low back and the sacroiliac joint on either side of your low back. Hold for two minutes or more. Repeat on the other side. Do this five or more times a day, reducing the repetitions as your symptoms start to subside. If this position hurts on one side, only do the side that feels good.

slacken the inside thighs (adductors; appendix i)

Most people sit with their legs and feet turned out to the sides. Sitting with your legs and feet slightly turned in will slacken the inside thigh muscles (adductors) and take strain off the lower back and the knees. Do not walk or stand in this position. Do this only when you are sitting. Do this every time you sit. Remember, this should not hurt. If it does, you are turning in your feet too far.

strengthen the inside thighs (adductors; appendix i)

Strengthening the adductor muscles will shorten the muscles on the inside of the upper leg and pull the legs back into alignment in a neutral position, taking the strain off the low back and knees. Do ten of these compressions and then rest for a minute and do ten more. Continue in this manner until you can do five sets of ten. This exercise will strengthen the muscles on the inside of your legs and begin to reduce your symptoms.

SUPPORTIVE LIFESTYLE: This part of your Wellness Plan is designed to address the root of the problem and to relieve habitual muscle imbalances to avoid aggravating the condition as you go about your daily life.

check sitting, driving, and computer positions (appendix a)

Correcting your posture while sitting, driving, and working at a computer will ensure the pelvis stays in balance and that you are not causing more stress on the neck, shoulders, and lower and upper back. These common activities are responsible for a great amount of the pain in your life. Doing these activities the incorrect way will make your body crooked and lead to muscle imbalances and possible lumbar or cervical disc problems. By slightly changing the way you sit, drive, and type on a computer, you will keep the body in alignment and help ensure that once the pain is relieved, it does not come back.

heat sore areas for twenty minutes

Use a heating pad on the sore areas every day for twenty minutes. Continue until the symptoms subside.

success story

A man in his forties came to see me who had suffered severe back pain for almost two years. He had a difficult time standing or sitting for long periods but had little or no pain when lying down. His doctor did an MRI of the region and found nothing unusual. This man sat at a desk all day for his work.

Most low back pain is simply due to muscle imbalances in the pelvic region, resulting in a crooked pelvis. Most people are crooked in three ways. This man certainly was when I measured him.

I performed three stretches to bring his pelvis back into balance and showed him how to do these stretches himself. I also showed him the proper sitting, computer, and driving positions that would help keep his pelvis straight.

He was a little nervous about getting off my table, because that movement for him was usually quite painful. Much to his surprise, he experienced only a little pain when getting off the table. He was already much improved.

I impressed upon him the importance of the Wellness Plan so that his pain would not return. The stretches in this chapter to balance the pelvis performed three times a day will help with most low back pain. He could not believe how simple it was to alleviate his pain after two years of suffering.

CHAPTER 13

IPT wellness plan for piriformis syndrome (sciatica)

The sciatic nerve has several branches coming out of the spinal cord into the lower back. Parts of the nerve run through the buttocks and down the back of each leg to the ankle and foot. When the sciatic nerve is irritated or compressed by a disc or a tight muscle, the condition is generally called sciatica. When this compression is caused by the piriformis muscle, it is called piriformis syndrome.

Piriformis syndrome and muscle-related sciatica are both caused by muscle imbalances in the hip and buttock muscles. Tight muscles are either too long or too short and pull or compress other structures in this area, leading to the pain. This condition is prevalent in people who sit improperly for long periods of time or do a lot of driving.

You can improve or eliminate muscle-related sciatica and piriformis syndrome with a little awareness and some self-care. It is vital to first identify and correct the common everyday activities that cause muscle strain that can lead to sciatica. Many activities you do every day may lead to pain and spasm in the muscles of the head, neck, shoulders, or back.

A logical first place to start is to make excellent posture a habit. Keeping your back rounded for long periods of time in your chair is a major cause of sciatic compressions. I believe that much of the sciatic pain in the country could be eliminated if everyone sat with the proper support. By correcting your computer and driving positions, you will bring your head over your shoulders and straighten out your back, giving yourself good posture and less pain.

It is very important that you perform the four stretches to balance the pelvis. These four stretches usually bring the pelvis back into alignment. The pelvis is commonly misaligned in three ways: 1) it is higher on one side; 2) it is rotated; 3) it is tilted either forward or backward. Most people have at least one of these imbalances, and many have all three. A balanced pelvis usually loosens the piriformis and takes the pressure off the sciatic nerve.

Although it is a common practice to stretch the piriformis, I have found that stretching this muscle will often aggravate sciatica. When you stretch a muscle, you temporarily make it tighter, like stretching a rubber band. This tightness then aggravates the nerve. Slackening usually feels good by taking pressure off the nerve. See the Wellness Plan for instructions for slackening the piriformis, which often brings dramatic relief along with instructions for slackening the hip flexors, another exercise that can bring quick relief from sciatic pain.

Lack of water can also be a factor in sciatic pain. Many people do not drink enough water to adequately hydrate their cells. Muscles that do not get enough water ache more than muscles that are well hydrated. Also, discs need to be well hydrated to maintain their softness and to prevent pinching or irritating a nerve. Good disc health is dependent on adequate water.

By adopting the Wellness Plan in this chapter, you can eliminate or significantly reduce your sciatica. If after practicing the Wellness Plan you still have no improvement, see your health care provider for further assessment.

symptoms:

Symptoms of piriformis syndrome or sciatica include pain that begins in your back or buttocks and moves down your leg and may move into your foot. Weakness, tingling, or numbness in the leg may also occur. These symptoms could indicate a disc problem or a tight piriformis. This condition is often worse when sitting or standing. Symptoms can range from mild to severe.

common causes:

Many lifestyle habits can contribute to sciatica. The following are some of the most common I have come across in my practice:

- Biking
- Sitting improperly
- Driving, especially a clutch

These activities can all cause muscle imbalances in the low back (lumbar region), which can lead to sciatica. Limiting these activities when you have sciatica will speed up the recovery process.

The following conditions caused by muscle imbalances are a major source of sciatica:

- Tight piriformis
- Herniated disc

These two physiological changes can also cause sciatica:

- Spinal stenosis
- Pregnancy

conventional medical approach

Standard medical treatments for sciatic pain often include painkillers, muscle relaxants, anti-depressants, cortisone, and anti-inflammatories. Physical therapy is also widely prescribed for this condition. Surgery is sometimes prescribed if these other measures are not working. Remember that drugs and surgery do not cure sciatica unless it is due to spinal stenosis or other bony or disc impingement on the sciatic nerve, which can be relieved surgically. Otherwise, drugs and surgery don't address one of the biggest factors of sciatica—muscle imbalances.

IPT wellness plan for piriformis syndrome (sciatica)

MUSCLE REBALANCING: This section provides the exercises you need to practice to correct the muscle imbalances causing your pain. By doing these exercises now and continuing to do them as instructed, you will make your short muscles longer and your long muscles shorter, bringing them back into balance.

four stretches to balance the pelvis (appendix b)

These stretches will help to bring the body structure back into balance, thus eliminating a major cause of aches and pains. These exercises are designed to stretch the muscles or muscle groups that are typically too short in most people and pull the pelvis out of alignment. When the pelvis is crooked, all the areas of the body are affected. A pelvis that is out of alignment is often a major cause of piriformis syndrome or sciatica. Do these stretches three times a day. Hold for one minute each.

half-frog (slacken the piriformis; appendix h)

The half-frog position will slacken the piriformis muscle and take strain off the sciatic nerve. Hold for two minutes or more. Repeat on the other side. Do this five or more times a day and less frequently as your symptoms start to subside. If this hurts on one side, only do the side that feels good.

slacken the hip flexors (psoas and quadriceps; appendix h)

The hip flexor muscles are typically too short in most people. The very act of sitting in a chair, which we have done our whole lives, makes the hip flexors short. These short hip flexors will pull the pelvis forward, resulting in an anterior pelvic tilt, which can cause an exaggerated curve in the low back and/or sciatica or disc problems. Slackening the hip flexors relaxes these muscles, allows the pelvis to return to neutral, and relieves pain.

slacken the inside thighs (adductors; appendix i)

Most people sit with their legs and feet turned out to the sides. Sitting with your legs and feet slightly turned in will slacken the adductors and gently release the piriformis, taking strain off the lower back and knees. Do not walk or stand like this. Do this only when you are sitting. Remember, this should not hurt. If it does, you are turning in your feet too far.

strengthen the inside thighs (adductors; appendix i)

Strengthening the adductor muscles will shorten the muscles on the inside of the upper leg and pull the legs back into neutral alignment so the strain is taken off the low back and the knees, releasing the piriformis. Do ten of these compressions, rest for a minute, and do ten more. Continue in this manner until you can do five sets of ten. This exercise will strengthen the muscles on the inside of your legs and begin to reduce your symptoms.

SUPPORTIVE LIFESTYLE: This part of your Wellness Plan is designed to address the root of the problem and to relieve habitual muscle imbalances to avoid aggravating the condition as you go about your daily life.

check sitting, driving, and computer positions (appendix a)

Correcting your posture while sitting, driving, and working at a computer will ensure the pelvis stays in balance and that you are not causing more stress on the neck, shoulders, and lower and upper back, which can compress the sciatic nerve and lead to sciatica or piriformis syndrome. These common activities are responsible for a great amount of the pain in your life. Sitting, driving, or typing on a computer the incorrect way will make your body crooked and lead to muscle imbalances and possible lumbar or cervical disc problems. By slightly changing the way you perform these activities, you will keep the body in alignment and help ensure that once the pain is relieved, it does not come back.

use heat on low back and buttocks

Use a heating pad on your low back and buttocks every day for twenty minutes. Continue until your symptoms subside.

success story

A man in his fifties came to see me who was suffering from sciatica. The pain was in his left buttock and traveled down the back of his left leg. He had suffered with this pain on and off for ten years. He had been to physical therapy many times with only moderate relief, but his doctor had given up on him.

What you do every day is almost always a major contributor to your aches and pains. I wanted to know what he did for a living. He said he was a truck driver. I asked him if his truck had a clutch. He said it did and stated that his pain was always worse when driving. I have seen this many times before. People usually have their foot on the clutch with the foot turned out, which in turn contracts the piriformis even more. In this man's case, this position was putting pressure on the sciatic nerve, sending pain down his leg.

I did the four stretches to balance the pelvis, which was quite crooked. I then had him lie facedown. When I pressed gently on his piriformis, the muscle was so tight and inflamed that he jumped and gave out a yelp. I immediately put him into the position known as half-frog, which will slacken the piriformis. I gently pressed the piriformis again. He said that the pain was gone. I pressed the piriformis a little harder and still he said he had no pain in the half-frog position.

I explained to him how crucial it was that he adapt the correct sitting and driving positions and that he needed to keep his foot on the clutch straight and not turned out. Before he got off my table, I told him he would still experience some pain because the nerve was irritated and inflamed.

I advised him that if he followed the Wellness Plan as described in this chapter, his pain would most likely be all gone in two to four weeks.

I saw him a month later and indeed his pain was gone. He remained pain-free as long as he used the proper lumbar support and kept his foot straight when using the clutch.

I encouraged him to keep performing the Wellness Plan, even though he felt better, so his sciatica would not return.

CHAPTER 14

IPT wellness plan for medial meniscus injury (knee pain)

The medial meniscus is a band of cartilage on the inside of the knee at the head of the tibia. There is also one on the outside of the knee. It is a common site of injury, especially in sports. The medial meniscus acts as a shock absorber between the tibia and the femur. Large tears to the meniscus may require surgery. Small tears will respond well to the protocols in this book. The meniscus is often damaged due to muscle imbalances in the hip and leg muscles. The tight muscles are either too long or too short and pull or compress the meniscus and other structures in this area, leading to pain.

Knee replacements have almost doubled in the last ten years. The truth is that your knees should last longer than you do. They will not wear out as long as your pelvis is straight and you have no underlying problem like rheumatoid arthritis. Think of our car example. If the front end of your car is out of alignment, your tires will wear out quickly. In this case, the tires are your knees. Keep the pelvis straight to save your knees. A straight pelvis will allow your knees to take the stress on them the way nature intended and last a long time.

You can improve or eliminate your knee pain with a little awareness and some self-care. It is vital to first identify and correct the common everyday activities that cause muscle strain in the pelvis and legs that can lead to pain in the knee.

One of the most common causes of these muscle imbalances is simply poor posture and/or improper ergonomics. Keeping your back rounded for long periods of time in your chair is a major cause of a crooked pelvis, which then leads to strain on the knees. I believe a great deal of the knee pain in the country could be eliminated if everyone sat with the proper support. By correcting your computer and driving positions, you will bring your head over your shoulders and straighten your back, giving yourself good posture. Your bones will be supporting you, which will take the strain off the knees.

Many people walk and sit with their feet turned out, which puts a lot of strain on the knee, especially on the inside (medial). It is important to correct the muscle imbalances that lead to walking this way. We need to train the feet to go back to the neutral position, which is pointing straight ahead. Try sitting with your toes slightly turned in. This position will often quickly take the strain off the knee and relieve the pain. Do not stand or walk with your toes turned in. Just sit that way.

When the feet are turned out, the muscles on the outside of the leg are too short. Doing the hip abductor stretch will lengthen those muscles and start to bring the feet straighter, which will often take the strain off the knee. Remember, this stretch should not hurt. If it does, you are turning in your feet too far.

Knee pain is also often caused by your quadriceps being too short. These are the muscles on the front of the upper leg that attach at the knee. Quadriceps that are too short can cause knee pain. Gently stretching these muscles will help to alleviate the pain.

Lack of water can also be a factor in knee pain. Muscles that do not get enough water ache more than muscles that are well hydrated. The knee joint needs to be well hydrated in order to be well lubricated, which will reduce or eliminate any inflammation in the knee. Good joint health is dependent on adequate water.

By adopting the Wellness Plan in this chapter, you can eliminate or significantly reduce your knee pain. If after practicing the Wellness Plan you still have no improvement, see your health care provider for further assessment.

symptoms:

Symptoms include pain on the inside of the knee, often accompanied by swelling. This can indicate anything from a sprain to a tear. The area is often painful to the touch. A person with medial meniscus injury may experience limited range of motion or popping and clicking sounds with movement, often accompanied by pain in the groin.

common causes:

Many lifestyle habits can contribute to knee pain. The following are some of the most common I have come across in my practice:

- Sports
- Dancing
- Driving
- Yoga
- Weightlifting
- Sitting with feet turned out

These activities can all cause muscle imbalances in the knee, which can lead to knee or medial meniscus pain. Limiting these activities when you have knee pain will speed up the recovery process.

The following conditions caused by muscle imbalances are a major source of knee pain:

- Imbalanced pelvis
- External rotators of the leg that are too short

conventional medical approach

Standard medical treatments for knee pain often include painkillers, muscle relaxants, hyaluronic acid injections, cortisone, and anti-inflammatories. Physical therapy is also widely prescribed for this condition. Surgery is sometimes prescribed if other measures are not working. Remember that drugs and surgery do not cure knee pain; rather, they alleviate the symptoms for a while. They do not address the primary cause of knee pain—muscle imbalances.

IPT wellness plan for medial meniscus injury (knee pain)

MUSCLE REBALANCING: This section provides the exercises you need to practice to correct the muscle imbalances that are causing your pain. By doing these exercises now and continuing to do them as instructed, you will make your short muscles longer and your long muscles shorter, bringing them back into balance.

four stretches to balance the pelvis (appendix b)

These stretches will help to bring the body structure back into balance, thus eliminating a major cause of aches and pains. These exercises are designed to stretch the muscles or muscle groups that are typically too short in most people and pull the pelvis out of alignment. When the pelvis is crooked, all the areas of the body are affected. A pelvis that is out of alignment is often a major cause of knee pain. Do these stretches three times a day. Hold for one minute each.

half-frog (slacken the piriformis; appendix h)

The half-frog position will slacken the piriformis muscle, allowing the leg and knee to return to a neutral position, taking strain off the knee. Hold the position for two minutes or more. Repeat on the other side. Do this five or more times a day and then less frequently as your symptoms start to subside. If this hurts on one side, only do the side that feels good.

slacken the hip flexors (psoas & quadriceps; appendix h)

The hip flexor muscles are typically too short in most people. The very act of sitting in a chair, which we have done our whole lives, makes the hip flexors short. These short hip flexors will pull the pelvis forward, resulting in an anterior pelvic tilt, which can cause an exaggerated curve in the low back. One of the hip flexors attaches near the knee and can put a lot of strain on the knee, a common condition. Slackening the hip flexors relaxes these muscles, allowing the pelvis to return to neutral and taking the strain off the knee.

slacken the inside thighs (adductors; appendix i)

Most people sit with their legs and feet turned out to the sides. Sitting with your legs and feet slightly turned in will take strain off the lower back and the knees. Do not walk or stand in this position. Do it only when you are sitting. Remember, this should not hurt. If it does, you are turning in your feet too far.

strengthen the inside thighs (adductors; appendix i)

After some healing occurs and your knee pain lessens, you can strengthen the adductors. Strengthening the adductors will shorten the muscles on the inside of the upper leg and pull the legs back into neutral alignment so that the strain is taken off the low back and the knees. Do ten of these compressions, rest for a minute, and do ten more. Continue in this manner until you can do five sets of ten. This exercise will strengthen the muscles on the inside of your legs and begin to reduce your symptoms.

SUPPORTIVE LIFESTYLE: This part of your Wellness Plan is designed to address the root of the problem and to relieve habitual muscle imbalances to avoid aggravating the condition as you go about your daily life.

check sitting, driving, and computer positions (appendix a)

Correcting your posture while sitting, driving, and working at the computer will ensure the pelvis stays in balance and that you are not placing more stress on the knees. These common activities are responsible for a great amount of the pain in your life. Doing these activities the wrong way will make your body crooked. By slightly changing the way you perform these activities, you will keep the body in alignment and help make sure that once the pain is relieved, it does not come back.

use heat on the quadriceps

The quadriceps are the muscles on the front part of the upper leg. Use a heating pad to warm the quadriceps twenty minutes every night. This will help to loosen those muscles and take strain off the knees.

success story

A woman in her sixties who was an avid yoga practitioner came to me complaining of moderate to severe knee pain in both knees. She had already had an operation to repair a tear in the medial meniscus on her left side. Now her doctor was telling her that she would probably need an operation on the other knee as well. Her doctor gave her some pain medication and she was going to physical therapy, which she said was making it worse.

She complained that the inside of her thighs, especially around the knee and groin, felt very tight. She was doing a lot of yoga stretches for that area but could not seem to get that tissue to feel loose no matter how much stretching she did.

I had her lie on her back and observed that her feet turned way out almost like a ballet dancer. In this condition, the tissue on the outside of the thigh is too short and tight, whereas the tissue on the inside of the thigh is too long and tight like an overstretched rubber band. I touched the inside of her knees and they were quite sore. I turned her legs and feet in for two minutes to rebalance those muscles affecting the knees. When I touched the tissue again, she had no pain. She could not believe it, as her knees had been sore for years.

Once I explained to her how the tissue was too long on the inside of her thighs and that stretching that tissue was making it worse, she understood.

I advised her to stop all stretching for the inside of the thigh (known in yoga as "hip openers"). I showed her how to strengthen the adductors and sit with the feet slightly turned in.

I showed her the four stretches to balance the pelvis and told her to do only those four stretches for about a month. She was not to stretch any other muscles.

Her knees recovered and she did not need an operation on her other knee. I stressed the importance of continuing the Wellness Plan to make sure her symptoms did not return.

CHAPTER 15

IPT wellness plan for plantar fasciitis (heel spur)

Plantar fasciitis is inflammation of the plantar fascia. This is the tissue that forms the arch of the foot. Plantar means bottom of the foot. Fascia is connective tissue, and -itis means inflammation.

A heel spur is a hook of bone that can form on the heel. Plantar fasciitis is often accompanied by a heel spur that can be seen on an X-ray. Heel spurs are soft, bendable deposits of calcium that are a result of mechanical tension and inflammation. Heel spurs usually do not cause pain. They are an indication that plantar fasciitis may be present, which is the real cause of the pain.

Plantar fasciitis condition is due to muscle imbalances in the pelvis, lower leg, and foot muscles. The tight muscles are either too long or too short and pull or compress other structures in this area, often leading to pain.

You can improve or eliminate your plantar fasciitis with a little awareness and some self-care. It is vital to first identify and correct the common everyday activities that are causing muscle strain in the pelvis, lower leg, and foot tissue that can lead to plantar fasciitis. Many activities you do every day may lead to pain and inflammation in these muscles.

As with most muscle imbalances, the first place to start is with proper posture. Keeping your back rounded for long periods of time in your chair is a major cause of a crooked pelvis, which then leads to strain on the feet and possibly plantar fasciitis.

Many people walk and sit with their feet turned out, which puts a lot of strain on the feet. It is important to correct the muscle imbalances that lead to walking this way. We need to train the feet to go back to the neutral position, which is pointing straight ahead. Try to sit with your toes turned in. Do not stand or walk with your toes turned in. Just sit that way. Remember, this should not hurt. If it does, you are turning in your feet too far.

The standard medical treatment for plantar fasciitis is to stretch the calf and ice the foot. I have found that this method may take months or years to heal the condition. A more effective treatment is to slacken the calf and foot as well as heat the foot by soaking it in warm water and Epsom salts every night. This will often bring relief in weeks not months.

If you have plantar fasciitis, wearing shoes with good arch supports is important. The arch support puts the bottom of the foot into slack and helps to relieve the pain. Walking barefoot or in flip-flops can aggravate plantar fasciitis.

Lack of water can also be a factor in plantar fasciitis. Muscles that do not get enough water ache more than muscles that are well hydrated. Water is a good anti-inflammatory.

By adopting the Wellness Plan in this chapter, you can eliminate or significantly reduce your plantar fasciitis. If after practicing the Wellness Plan you still have no improvement, see your health care provider for further assessment.

symptoms:

With plantar fasciitis the most common complaint is pain in the bottom of the heel or other part of the plantar area. It is usually worse in the morning and improves throughout the day. It often occurs in conjunction with a tight, sore calf and/or Achilles tendon.

common causes:

Many lifestyle habits can contribute to plantar fasciitis. The following are some of the most common I have come across in my practice:

- Long periods of standing or walking
- Running
- Dancing
- Wearing improper shoes

These activities can all cause muscle imbalances in the calf and foot, which can lead to plantar fasciitis. Limiting these activities when you have plantar fasciitis will speed up the recovery process. Wear shoes that have good arch supports.

The following conditions caused by muscle imbalances are a major source of plantar fasciitis:

- Imbalanced hip
- Tight calf
- Tight Achilles tendon
- Flat feet

conventional medical approach

Standard medical treatments for plantar fasciitis often include painkillers, muscle relaxants, cortisone, and anti-inflammatories. Physical therapy is also widely prescribed for this condition. Orthotics and a night splint that keeps the calf stretched all night are common prescriptions. Surgery is sometimes prescribed if other measures are not working. Remember that drugs and surgery do not always cure plantar fasciitis; rather, they alleviate the symptoms for a while. They do not address the primary cause of plantar fasciitis—muscle imbalances.

IPT wellness plan for plantar fasciitis (heel spur)

MUSCLE REBALANCING: This section provides the exercises you need to practice to correct the muscle imbalances causing your pain. By doing these exercises now and continuing to do them as instructed, you will make your short muscles longer and your long muscles shorter, bringing them back into balance.

four stretches to balance the pelvis (appendix b)

These stretches will help to bring the body structure back into balance, thus eliminating a major cause of aches and pains. These exercises are designed to stretch the muscles or muscle groups that are typically too short in most people and pull the pelvis out of alignment. A crooked pelvis affects all the areas of the body. A pelvis that is out of alignment is often a major cause of plantar fasciitis. Do these stretches three times a day and hold for one minute each.

achilles tendon release (appendix j)

The Achilles tendon is the thick cord on the back of the heel that attaches the calf to the heel. Releasing this tendon takes the strain off the calf and the plantar area (bottom of the foot.). Hold the position for two minutes and repeat the exercise three times a day.

slacken the calf (appendix j)

Slackening the calf releases the calf muscle and the Achilles tendon and gives almost immediate relief. Hold the position for two minutes. Do this exercise at least five times a day. In this case, the more often you slacken the calf, the better.

gentle stretching of calf muscles (appendix j)

Gently stretching the calf will lengthen the muscle and takes the strain off the bottom of the foot. Do not stretch too deeply. Stretching deeply can aggravate plantar fasciitis. If stretching hurts, the stretch is too deep. Repeat five to ten times a day and less frequently as the pain starts to subside.

strengthen the inside thighs (adductors; appendix i)

Strengthening the adductor muscles will shorten the muscles on the inside of the upper leg and pull the legs back into alignment to remove strain from the low back and knees. When your legs are in their neutral position, your feet will strike the ground as nature intended when you are walking, helping to alleviate plantar fasciitis. Do ten of the compressions, rest for a minute, and do ten more. Continue in this manner until you can do five sets of ten.

slacken the inside thighs (adductors; appendix i)

Most people sit with their legs and feet turned out to the sides. Sitting with your legs and feet slightly turned in will train your body to walk with your feet straight and thus take the strain off the plantar fascia. Do not walk or stand in this position. Do this only when you are sitting. Remember, this should not hurt. If it does, you are turning in your feet too far.

SUPPORTIVE LIFESTYLE: This part of your Wellness Plan is designed to address the root of the problem and to relieve habitual muscle imbalances to avoid aggravating the condition as you go about your daily life.

check sitting, driving, and computer positions (appendix a)

Correcting your posture while sitting, driving, and working at the computer will ensure the pelvis stays in balance and that you are not causing more stress on the plantar fascia and Achilles tendon. These common activities are responsible for a great amount of the pain in your life. Doing these activities the incorrect way will make your body crooked. By slightly changing the way you perform these activities, you will keep the body in alignment and help make sure that once the pain is relieved, it does not come back.

proper arch support

Walking barefoot aggravates plantar fasciitis. Always wear shoes with good arch supports. Good arch supports keep the calf muscles and the bottom of the foot in slack. Fortunately, most of the brand names have good arch support. Athletic shoes are best. Avoid sandals and flip-flops until your pain goes away.

rest

If you are a runner or are on your feet a lot, good old-fashioned rest will be quite helpful. Rest is still nature's great healer. The more you can rest, the quicker you will see results.

soak your feet in epsom salts and warm water

Soak your feet in a little tub of warm water for twenty minutes a night for five nights. Make the water deep enough to cover your Achilles tendon. Use about one pound of Epsom salts to three to five gallons of water. Epsom salt is magnesium sulfate, a natural muscle relaxant and anti-inflammatory.

success story

A man in his thirties came to me who he had been diagnosed with plantar fasciitis. X-rays showed he also had a heel spur. He had sharp pain on the bottom of his heel when standing or walking. He had been a runner but had not been able to run for the previous eight months because of the pain. His doctor had given him a cortisone shot, which helped for a couple of weeks. He was going to physical therapy, which was only helping a little. He was also wearing a boot at night that kept his calf and Achilles tendon stretched all night. He stated that the pain was 8 on a scale of 10.

I have treated many cases of plantar fasciitis, and I know that the standard medical approach seldom brings the desired results. With him lying facedown on my table, I pressed the spot on his heel where the pain was located. He reported that it was quite painful. I put him in the "slacken the calf" position and pressed the spot again. He said it was still sore but much less so. I held that position for two minutes and then pressed the spot again. He said he now felt no pain. He couldn't believe it could be that easy!

He wanted to know if he could start running again.

I explained to him that although he felt better, he still had some inflammation and that the pain would return if he did not follow the Wellness Plan to rebalance his muscles. I told him that after he rebalanced his muscles and the inflammation decreased by 70%, he could slowly start running again.

On a follow-up visit, he reported that he had started running two weeks after he last saw me and had been running ever since. I encouraged him to continue to follow the Wellness Plan so his symptoms would not return.

CHAPTER 16

IPT wellness plan for fibromyalgia

Fibromyalgia means pain in the muscles, ligaments, and tendons—the soft tissues in the body. Fibromyalgia is a chronic condition that also presents as fatigue and multiple tender points. Tender points can be found in the back of the neck, shoulders, chest, lower back, hips, elbows, and knees. The pain may spread from these areas. These tender points will be on both the left and right side of the body and both above and below the waist.

This condition is often due to muscle imbalances in many different muscles all over the body. Tight muscles are either too long or too short and pull or compress other structures in the body, leading to pain.

People with fibromyalgia tend to wake up with body aches and stiffness, often because they have not consumed any water all night. Fibromyalgia is more common in women than in men. Other names for this condition are fibrositis, chronic muscle pain syndrome, and tension myalgias.

You can improve or eliminate your fibromyalgia with a little awareness and some self-care. It is vital to first identify and correct the common everyday activities that cause muscle strain in the neck, shoulders, upper and lower back, and arms and legs that can lead to fibromyalgia. Many activities you do every day may lead to widespread pain and spasm in the muscles in various parts of the body.

One of the most common causes of these muscle imbalances is simply poor posture and/or improper ergonomics, which then leads to strain in widespread areas of the body that could be diagnosed as fibromyalgia. By correcting your computer and driving positions, you will bring your head over your shoulders and straighten your back, giving yourself good posture. Your bones (the spinal column) will be supporting you, which will take the strain off the muscles and reduce or eliminate the pain.

Lack of water can also be a factor in fibromyalgia. Many people do not drink enough water to adequately hydrate their cells. Muscles that do not get enough water ache more than muscles that are well hydrated. I have observed that many of the people who come to me with a diagnosis of fibromyalgia are dehydrated to a greater or lesser degree.

By adopting the Wellness Plan in this chapter, you can eliminate or significantly reduce your widespread pain. If after practicing the Wellness Plan you still have no improvement, see your health care provider for further assessment.

symptoms:

Fibromyalgia is characterized by chronic, widespread pain with tenderness to light touch. The pain can be mild to severe and is often accompanied by fatigue. The skin often tingles in a way that feels like needles. Nerve pain, brain fog, and trouble sleeping are common as well.

common causes:

There is no known cause of fibromyalgia, but the following are significant contributors:

- Postural deviations
- Improper sitting posture
- Improper driving positions
- Improper computer positions

These activities can all cause muscle imbalances in the body, which can lead to fibromyalgia. Limiting or correcting these activities will speed up the recovery process.

The following habits lead to chemical imbalances in the body, muscle pain, and fatigue:

- Lack of water
- Too much caffeine
- Poor diet

conventional medical approach

Standard medical treatments for fibromyalgia often include painkillers, muscle relaxants, anti-depressants, anti-seizure drugs, and anti-inflammatories. Remember that the drugs do not cure fibromyalgia; rather, they alleviate the symptoms for a while. They do not address one of the biggest causes of fibromyalgia—muscle imbalances.

IPT wellness plan for fibromyalgia

MUSCLE REBALANCING: This section provides the exercises you should practice to correct the muscle imbalances that are causing your pain. By doing these exercises now and continuing to do them as instructed, you will make your short muscles longer and your long muscles shorter, bringing them back into balance.

four stretches to balance the pelvis (appendix b)

These stretches will help to bring the body structure back into balance, thus eliminating a major cause of aches and pains. These exercises are designed to stretch the muscles or muscle groups that are typically too short in most people and pull the pelvis out of alignment. When the pelvis is crooked, all areas of the body are affected. A pelvis that is out of alignment is often a factor in fibromyalgia. Do these stretches three times a day. Hold each stretch for one minute.

three neck stretches (appendix c)

Gently stretch the neck muscles three times a day. Loosening the muscles in the neck and shoulders will allow more blood and oxygen to flow to the head and neck. It takes a few minutes to stretch these muscles. It is a great habit to cultivate, as you will feel less pain and stiffness in the neck and will be more alert. Consistent practice will reduce or eliminate the cause of your neck pain and may help with "brain fog."

slacken the shoulders (levator scapula & upper trapezius; appendix e)

Slackening the shoulders will relieve tension in the shoulders, especially the upper traps and levator scapula. These areas are tight and sore in most people. Hold the position for at least two minutes. Do this exercise anytime you feel tension in your shoulders or neck and at least five times each day. Do not do this exercise if it hurts to put your arm on top of your head.

stretch the chest (pectoralis major & minor; appendix f)

In most people the chest muscles are too short and the rhomboids between the shoulder blades are too long, which gives a person a head-forward, bent-over look with rounded shoulders. Stretching the chest muscles will release tension between the shoulder blades and open up the chest, which will make a person stand up straighter. When a person stands straight, the bones in the cervical spine support the head, and the neck muscles can relax. Hold the positions for at least two minutes, and do the exercise two to four times a day.

slacken the chest (appendix f)

Slackening the chest will relax the muscles in the chest, especially the pectoralis minor muscle. Relaxing these muscles helps people with shoulders rounded forward to bring them back into better alignment and will help bring the head over the shoulder, reducing strain on the neck. Totally relax and hold the position for two minutes.

slacken the calf (appendix j)

Slackening the calf releases the calf muscle and the Achilles tendon. Do this exercise at least five times a day. Hold for two minutes. In this case, more often is better.

gentle stretching of calf muscles (appendix j)

Stretching the calf will lengthen the muscle and relieve the pain in that area. Do not stretch too deeply. If this hurts, the stretch is too deep. Do this five to ten times a day and then less frequently as the pain starts to subside. Hold for one minute.

strengthen the inside thighs (adductors; appendix i)

Strengthening the adductor muscles will shorten the muscles on the inside of the upper leg and pull the legs back into neutral alignment so that the strain is taken off the low back and knees. Do ten of the compressions, rest for a minute, and do ten more. Continue in this manner until you can do five sets of ten. This exercise will strengthen the muscles on the inside of your legs and begin to reduce your symptoms.

slacken the inside thighs (adductors; appendix i)

Most people sit with their legs and feet turned out to the sides. Sitting with your legs and feet slightly turned in will take strain off the lower back and the knees. Do not walk or stand in this position. Do this only when you are sitting. Remember, this should not hurt. If it does, you are turning in your feet too far.

SUPPORTIVE LIFESTYLE: This part of your Wellness Plan is designed to address the root of the problem and to relieve habitual muscle imbalances to avoid aggravating the condition as you go about your daily life.

check sitting, driving, and computer positions (appendix a)

Correcting your posture while sitting, driving, and working at the computer will ensure the pelvis stays in balance and that you are not causing more stress on the neck, shoulders, and lower and upper back that can lead to fibromyalgia symptoms. These common activities are responsible for a great amount of the pain in your life. Doing these activities the incorrect way will make your body crooked. By slightly changing the way you perform these activities, you will keep the body in alignment and ensure that once the pain is relieved, it does not come back.

keep well hydrated

One of the most common causes of widespread pain is dehydration. Even slight dehydration can cause muscle aches and cramps. Many people are dehydrated. If you have fibromyalgia, start hydrating as soon as possible. See chapter 17 for instructions on how to drink water and how much. It can take up to six weeks to rehydrate.

epsom salt bath

Soak your body in a tub of warm water for twenty minutes. Use four pounds of Epsom salts every night for five nights. Epsom salt is magnesium sulfate, a natural muscle relaxant and anti-inflammatory.

heat sore areas for twenty minutes

Use a heating pad on sore areas every day for twenty minutes. The heat will help the muscles relax and feel better. Continue this treatment until symptoms subside.

success story

A thirty-year-old woman came to me with a diagnosis from her doctor of fibromyalgia. She was in constant pain over most of her body; her muscles and especially her joints were very sore. Depending on the day, her pain levels were anywhere between 6 and 8 on a scale of 10. She was having trouble remembering things and was also experiencing depression. Her doctor had prescribed painkillers and antidepressants. She reported experiencing this pain for the last five years.

When I touched her muscles, it was obvious to me that she was dehydrated. Her muscles did not feel like well-hydrated tissue. Her posture was quite poor, which indicated numerous muscle imbalances. It took me about thirty minutes to rebalance her muscles and bring her body back into alignment. Her pain levels decreased immediately. I explained to her that her pain would not completely go away until her tissues were rehydrated. Improved fluid intake would most likely also help with her depression and brain fog. I explained that it could take up to six weeks to rehydrate.

I showed her the Wellness Plan and instructed her to be consistent, doing the plan every day so her muscle imbalances would not return. I also gave her advice on how to rehydrate her body.

I saw her two months later and she reported she felt greatly improved, although she still had some pain. Sometimes the rehydration and the Wellness Plan take a little longer to work.

Another month after that, she reported being 90% pain-free. She said that many days she had no pain at all. She also told me she had stopped taking painkillers and antidepressants and that her mood had greatly improved.

CHAPTER 17

the basic care of your body

Your body is much like your car. As long as you are using it, it requires some maintenance. I have culled from my practice the most effective habits to cultivate so you can thrive. When practiced consistently, you will have more energy and less pain.

In this chapter, you will find:

- simple practices to help increase your water and oxygen levels
- the daily 5 for better posture and less pain
- an easy practice to dramatically lower your stress levels, which will help you live pain-free

In order for the body to function at peak health, you must consume two vital "nutrients" in adequate amounts. These are oxygen and water. Usually we don't give these much thought, but they are involved in almost every function of the body. Without these two nutrients, life cannot exist. Pain levels are usually much higher when these two nutrients are not in adequate supply. When your body has enough oxygen and water, then the next step is for the nutrient to get to the cells. This task is done through circulation. Exercise is, of course, the best way to increase your circulation so your cells can receive all that life-giving, pain-reducing oxygen and water.

oxygen

If you ask people what is the most important ingredient for good health, you will seldom receive the right answer. The most common answers are plenty of water or nutritious food. Both of those are important, but not nearly as important as oxygen. Think about it. People can live thirty days with no food and still will not die. People can live five days with no water and still be alive. However, five minutes without oxygen causes death. Clearly oxygen is the most important factor in achieving good health and a pain-free body. Everything in the body works better when it receives an adequate supply of oxygen.

Many people do not get enough oxygen. This is mainly due to the fact that we breathe shallowly. By that, I mean we are using only a small part of our lungs. This is what is referred to as chest breathing. Proper breathing by using all of the lungs starts with the abdominal area filling up with air and then the chest. Most people fill up only the chest, which is about a third of our lung capacity. This amount will keep you alive but does not provide enough oxygen for optimal health.

Another reason we do not get enough oxygen is that our air does not contain as much oxygen as it once did. When scientists measure the percentage of oxygen in the air in a pristine environment, such as a country setting with lots of trees and few cars, the measurement of oxygen today tends to be in the mid 20% range. When they measure the oxygen content in an air sample from a big city with few trees and many cars, the oxygen percentage is in the mid-teens. Oxygen samples from inside buildings are even lower. They can be as low as 10%.

What is even more eye-opening is that the oxygen content measured from ice samples from three thousand years ago show the oxygen content of the air bubbles of that time to be 40%. As we continue to cut down trees and pollute the air, we are slowly depriving ourselves of the most vital nutrient on the planet.

Aside from keeping us alive, why is oxygen so important? Low levels of oxygen are associated with all sorts of chronic diseases. Oxygen helps to clean the blood of bacteria and viruses. Oxygen gives you more energy and boosts the immune system. Higher levels of oxygen are usually accompanied by better overall heath.

Eighty percent of all the pain people experience in their lives is muscular pain caused by muscle imbalances. The reason that not every tight muscle causes pain has to do with the amount of oxygen the tissues are receiving. When tissues do not get adequate oxygen, they hurt a lot more than tissue that is getting enough oxygen. Even if you have a tight muscle, as long as you are getting sufficient oxygen, the oxygen will reduce or eliminate the pain.

The easiest way to get more oxygen is to develop a daily practice of deep, slow breathing. This is easy to do and has many benefits, such as reduced pain levels, clearer thinking, more energy, reduced blood pressure, and lower stress levels. Do the following exercise at least twice a day for ten to fifteen minutes and also for shorter durations during the day. It may take some practice to break the habit of chest breathing, but it is well worth the effort.

daily practice:

- Sit up straight or lie on your back.
- Place a hand on your abdomen and slowly inhale through your nose.
- As you inhale, make sure that you feel your abdomen expanding against your hand.
- After your abdomen is full, continue to inhale. Now you should feel your chest expanding. This should be done with no effort or straining.
- Slowly exhale through your nose or mouth.
- Repeat the process.

water

Water is critical for all body functions. Experts agree that the body is 60–70% water. Many people are dehydrated—not clinically dehydrated, but enough to cause some serious problems. Proper hydration is the key to all of the body's critical systems. Good health is almost impossible if your cells are not hydrated properly. Signs of dehydration include fatigue, dizziness, constipation, arthritis, headaches, high blood pressure, anxiety, and dark-colored urine.

Water is so important that one of the first procedures a doctor will do when you are admitted to the hospital is to give you intravenous saline solution to help you quickly hydrate. Doctors know that good hydration is crucial to good health and reduced muscle pain.

We lose a lot of water simply through breathing. If you are out on a cold day, you can see the water vapor with every breath. If you live in a cold climate and live in a heated house, the typical humidity is 15–20%. That is considered desert conditions. Breathing dry air can lead to dehydration.

Remember that caffeine and alcohol are diuretics and thus take water out of the body. These types of drinks will not hydrate but rather dehydrate and should be consumed in moderation. Drink a little extra water after consuming drinks with caffeine or alcohol.

As the body starts to get low on water, it has to manage this crisis. The body has a priority system as to how it uses its water. The main priority is the brain. The body does not want the brain to get low on water. If the body is not getting enough water, it has to take it from other places to send to the brain to keep it functioning well.

One of the places the body takes the water from is the joints. As a result, the joints will not be lubricated enough, which will cause them to ache and be painful. The body also takes water from the discs between the vertebrae. This can cause the body to get shorter and possibly compress a nerve, which is very painful. The body also takes water from the muscles to send to the brain. This reallocation can cause the muscles to ache more and be less flexible. When the body can no longer get enough water to send to the brain, symptoms such as memory loss, brain fog, and headaches can occur.

How much water and fluids should a person consume every day? The key is not how much you drink but how much your cells absorb. This amount can depend on many factors. In general:

- Water is better absorbed when it is sipped slowly and not guzzled.
- It is also better absorbed when it is room temperature, warm, or hot.
- If you are not on a salt-restricted diet, you will also absorb more water if you add a pinch of sea salt or Himalayan salt to the water. The minerals in the salt let the cells take in more water.
- Coconut water is also excellent for rehydrating the body.
- Sea salt and coconut water both contain electrolytes, which are vital minerals that are lost through sweat and urine. Electrolytes need to be replenished daily, as they are vital to hydration.

daily practice:

- Have a glass of room temperature water upon awakening to replace the fluids lost during sleep.
- Sip water or herbal tea all day long.
- Replenish your electrolytes daily.
- Carry a water bottle with you when you are not home so you have a supply of water.
- Be consistent. It takes up to six weeks to rehydrate.
- Try to consume half of your body weight in ounces of water. For example, if you weigh 150 pounds, try consuming 75 oz. of fluid a day. Build up to these levels slowly so as not to overtax your bodily systems.
- If you are taking a diuretic, check with you doctor first before rehydrating.

exercise

It is well known that people who exercise are usually healthier and have more energy. One of the reasons for their superior health is that they are getting more water and oxygen to their cells through increased blood flow. Blood delivers oxygen and water to the cells, which increases energy and decreases pain.

Exercise raises your heart rate. The heart is the pump that circulates your blood. The better the circulation, the more energy you have and the less pain you experience. Even if you have sore muscles, often just a twenty-minute walk will raise the heart rate enough to reduce pain. If you are not able to walk for that long, find other ways to increase your heart rate. Start with five minutes and work up from there.

Exercise also contributes to better mental focus and a reduced chance of suffering from depression. Exercise stimulates brain chemicals that can make you happier and more relaxed. Exercise also helps to prevent or reverse osteoporosis. It will also improve your digestion, increase your metabolism, and help you to sleep better. Exercise helps to manage cholesterol and helps to prevent Type 2 diabetes. With all these benefits, it is certainly worthwhile to include some exercise in your daily life.

Many people lead a sedentary life. They wake up in the morning, drive to work, sit at work all day, drive home, watch TV, and then go to bed. That is a recipe for painful, weak, unbalanced muscles, depression and/or brain fog, unhealthy weight levels, and sleepless nights. The old adage "use it or lose it" is true. Before exercising, of course check with your doctor and see if you are fit to do so. There is no need for fancy equipment or expensive gyms, although those are fine. Simple walking will do. The human body was designed to walk many miles a day back when we were hunter-gatherers. Start with just ten minutes of walking a day if that is where your fitness level feels comfortable. The main thought to keep in mind is not to do too much too soon. Moderation is the key. Daily exercise that raises your heart rate even a little will bring tremendous benefits to your physical and mental state of being.

daily practice:

- Walk or do some gentle exercise that raises the heart rate for twenty to thirty minutes a day. This could be spread out to ten minutes three times a day.
- Rebounding on a mini trampoline is also an excellent form of exercise that is easy on the joints.
- Increase the time slowly as your fitness level improves.

the daily 5 for better posture and less pain

In my private practice, I consistently recommend four stretches and one strengthening exercise to my clients. Most people will benefit from practicing these exercises in addition to the exercises for your particular condition. Make them a part of your daily routine, and you will be training your muscles to give you better posture and less pain. You will also have more energy and be able to think more clearly.

This routine is also appropriate even if you have no pain at all. Make sure you are not stretching too deeply. If it hurts, you are stretching too deeply.

daily practice:

- Stretch the quads (see Appendix B).
- Stretch the psoas (see Appendix B).
- Stretch the hip abductors (see Appendix B).
- Stretch the chest (see Appendix F).
- Strengthen the hip extensors (see Appendix H).

These should be done two to five times a day for best results. It doesn't take very long.

meditation and pain relief

The benefits of meditation for pain relief are many. Chronic pain affects a staggering one hundred million Americans each year. Many people have been suffering with their pain for several years.

I have noticed that my clients have often tried many different approaches to help themselves with their pain. They take up an exercise program, change their diets, and start taking nutritional supplements. These can often bring some relief, but it has been my experience that sometimes diets, supplements, and exercise can only take you to a certain stage. Few of my clients have ever told me that they have tried meditation for pain relief.

Numerous medical schools like Harvard, Yale, and UCLA have conducted studies that prove a consistent meditation practice provides significant benefits to those who suffer from chronic pain, stress, and anxiety. Many of these studies can be found in well-respected publications such as *The Journal of Pain, The Journal of Neuroscience,* and *The Journal of the American Medical Association.* Lowering brain wave frequencies through meditation can bring dramatic and long-lasting relief from pain, stress, and anxiety, but this will require consistent practice.

Neuroscientists believe that stress reduction is a major component of meditation's beneficial effect on our health. From a muscular viewpoint, emotional stress, which causes a "fight or flight" condition in the body by releasing adrenaline into the system, will make the muscles in the body tighter and more painful. Many of the common diseases in America, such as hypertension and cardiac issues, have stress as a major component. Studies have also shown that people diagnosed with fibromyalgia (widespread pain in the body) have improved by practicing meditation. A person can achieve lower stress levels in as little as four to six weeks of a regular meditation practice.

daily practice:

- Meditation on the Breath
- Sit comfortably in a chair with a pillow in the small of your back (see Appendix A). This is an easy and comfortable way to sit.
- Gently close your eyes.
- Bring your attention to the breath. Do not try to control it. Simply observe the breath moving in and out of the lungs.
- Undoubtedly the mind will wander and begin thinking other thoughts. When this happens, gently bring your attention back to watching the breath.
- Start by practicing five to ten minutes a day. You will soon find that you can focus more easily and feel more relaxed.

thank you

I want to personally thank you for your dedication and commitment to your own individual self-care and for taking your care and compassion out into the world. By sharing the ideas in this book, many people will be able to help each other have less pain and more vitality.

We are at a time in the world when traditional medical models often have no long-term solutions for what we feel in our bodies. We are seeking solutions that offer more than short-term relief. Intuitively, we feel a need for the knowledge that can help us heal ourselves. We feel a need to learn how to be less stressed without drugs and how to have happiness as we journey through life. I have been helping people for over thirty years to achieve a pain-free life. It has been my experience that the IPT protocols discussed in this book have given many the knowledge to have more ease in their bodies and more calm in their hearts.

We all have a hand in weaving a new future for the world. Together, we are making a difference! I believe we are on this planet to help each other. There can be no greater aspiration than to help your family, friends, and neighbors achieve a more fulfilling life by having less pain and stress, and more peace and happiness. The Dalai Lama said it best: "When we feel love and kindness toward others, it not only makes others feel loved and cared for, but it helps us also to develop inner happiness and peace."

It is my utmost desire that the information contained in this book will be of some value on your journey while you are on this planet. Try what I have suggested and see for yourself that you are capable of helping yourself lead a more fulfilling life. I wish you much peace, happiness, and of course a pain-free life.

acknowledgments

I would like to take this opportunity to gratefully acknowledge the work of some amazing people whose contributions were invaluable.

To Marcia Albert, my wife, who so willingly gave of her time to read the manuscript and was able to figure out what I was really trying to say and then help me choose the right words.

To Lisa Oliver, MD, who read through the manuscript and made sure that I was medically accurate and helped me navigate medical terms and protocols.

To my models Andy Steigmeier LMT, CSCS, and Laura Jensen for never complaining when we had to shoot the same photo over and over to make me happy.

To my photographer Karla Archambeault, who made sure every detail of the photos was correct and kept everyone happy and on track.

To my illustrator Philip Nato, who redrew everything without a single complaint until I figured out what I really wanted.

I give each of you a heartfelt thank you for your love, support, and expertise. Your contributions have meant everything to me.

—Lee Albert, NMT

For more information, please visit Lee's website at
www.LeeAlbert.com

caution

With the following exercises, never stretch into a painful position. You will achieve better results by being gentle.

The goal is not to stretch as far as possible but to slightly increase range of motion. Done consistently, the results can be dramatic and permanent. Nothing should ever hurt while doing these exercises.

If pain occurs during an exercise, try the stretch or position more gently. If it still hurts, skip that exercise for now and continue with the ones that don't hurt.

If you are not getting better in three to five months of doing these protocols, please check with your health care provider for more insight into your condition.

appendices

appendix a 134

appendix b 137

appendix c 141

appendix d 143

appendix e 144

appendix f 146

appendix g 147

appendix h 149

appendix i 150

appendix j 151

appendix a
Proper Sitting, Driving, and Computer Positions

Proper Sitting Position	
Sit with a pillow placed in the lumbar curve. This is just above the belt line. It is important that the pillow is the right thickness. Every chair and every body needs a different thickness. The pillow should be thick enough to bring your head back over your shoulders and open the chest. A pillow that is too thick will be uncomfortable, and if it is not thick enough, your head will be forward of your body. The correct position allows the skeleton to support your body and should feel comfortable. This will contribute to overall good posture and reduced back and neck pain. If this is painful, disregard for now.	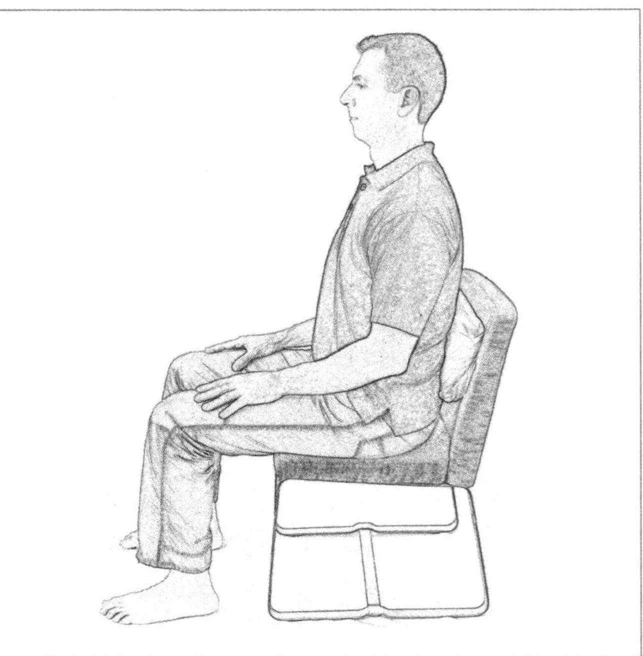

Improper Sitting Position	
This typical unsupported position can cause muscle tension in the low back, upper back, neck, and shoulders. This position can also make the hips uneven and lead to disc problems. In this position, your muscles are working to hold you up, creating tension and pain.	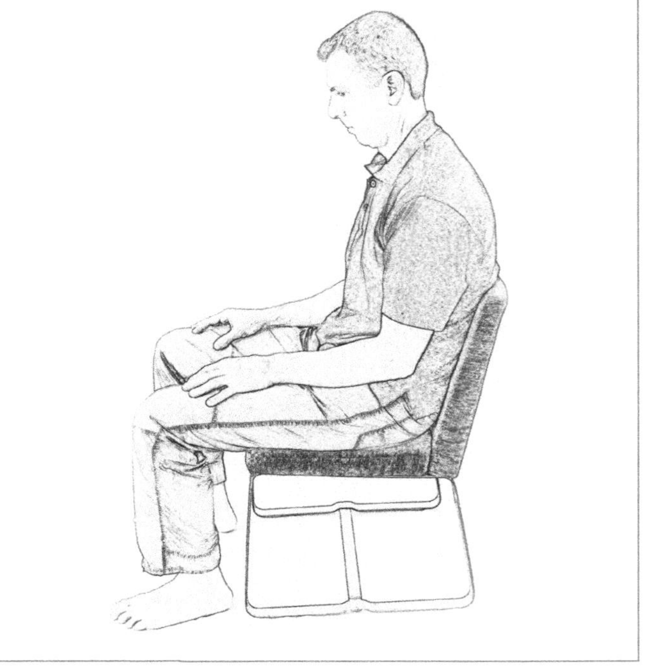

Proper Computer Position	
When sitting at your desk, keep your elbows by your side. Arms should be bent about 90 degrees. To find this position, stand normally with your arms at your side. Bend the elbows to 90 degrees. That should be how it looks and feels when you are sitting. The computer monitor should be eye level and straight in front of you so you are not bending your neck. Feet should be on the floor or on a foot rest and slightly turned in. Dangling feet can cause low back pain and poor circulation.	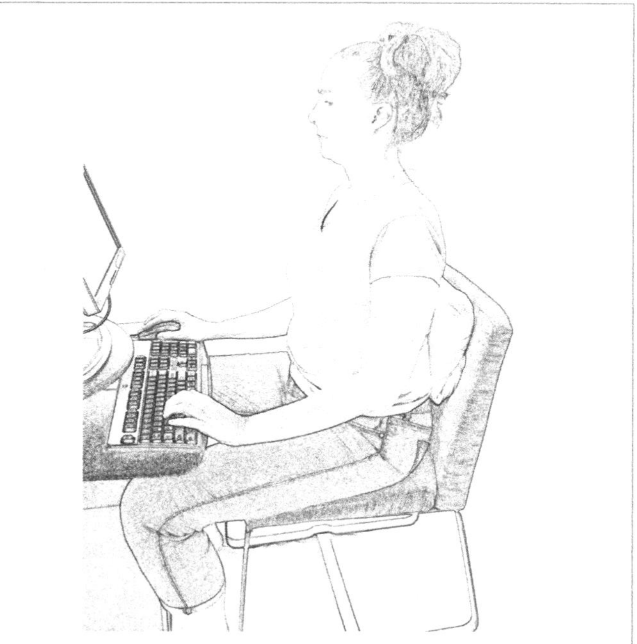

Improper Computer Position	
This common position can cause muscle tension in the jaw, shoulder, and neck. Do not reach for the mouse or keyboard.	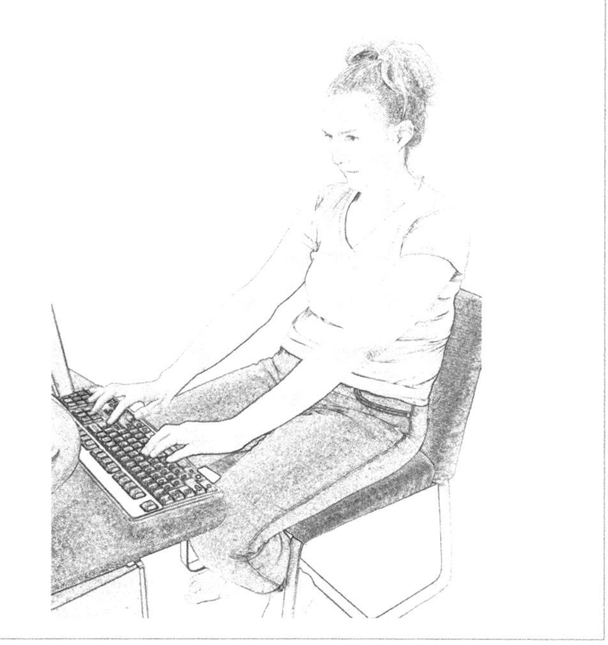

Proper Driving Position

When driving, use your pillow and keep your elbows at your side. Hands should be at the eight o'clock and four o'clock positions. This position allows your bones to support your body, avoids excessive muscle tension in the neck and shoulders, and helps to avoid potential trauma to the face if your air bags deploy. Many states now teach their new drivers to hold the wheel at eight and four as a safety precaution to prevent injury from airbag deployment.

WARNING: If you do not feel safe driving at the four o'clock and eight o'clock hand positions, then drive the way you normally do. It is better to have sore muscles and be safe. If you do feel comfortable driving at four and eight, you will find that this is a much better ergonomic position.

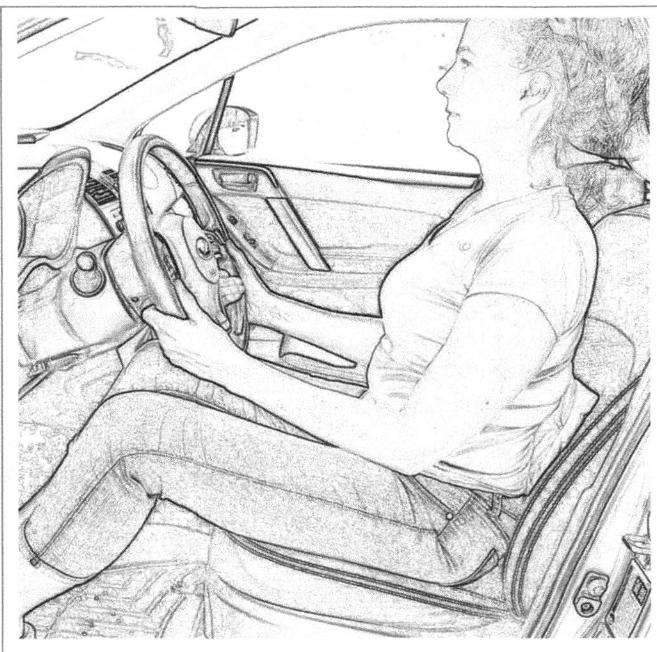

Improper Driving Position

Driving with hands at the ten o'clock and two o'clock positions can cause muscle tension in the upper back, shoulders, and neck.

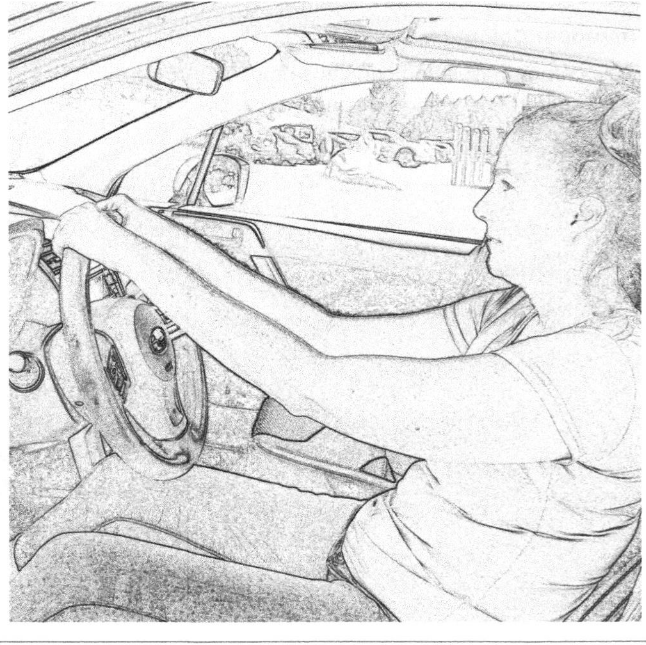

appendix b
four stretches to balance the pelvis

These stretches will usually bring your pelvis into alignment. They will ensure there is no abnormal strain on your hip joints, knees, or feet, and they correct the most common imbalances in the pelvis. Perform these four stretches three times per day to keep your hips in alignment. Hold these stretches for one minute. These stretches should be done gently and should not cause any pain. Breathe normally throughout these exercises; don't hold your breath!

Quadratus Lumborum Stretch	
Stand up straight with your legs slightly apart. Raise your arms and slowly bend toward the one side, reaching until you feel a stretch along the side of your upper body. Hold one minute. Repeat on the other side.	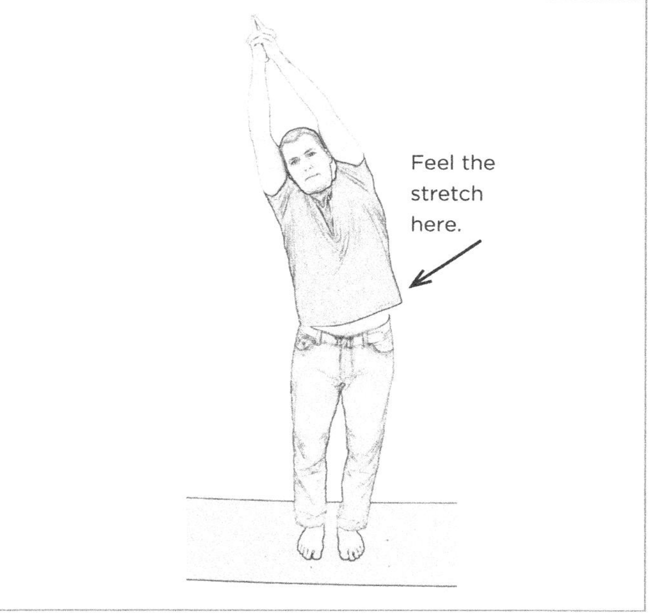

Quadratus Lumborum Stretch (modified)	
Stand up straight with your legs slightly apart. Raise your arm on one side so that your fingers are pointing toward the ceiling. Rest your forearm on top of your head. On the side where the arm is on your head, slowly bend toward the opposite side, until you feel a stretch along the side of your upper body. Rest the non-reaching hand on your leg. Hold one minute while breathing normally. Repeat on the other side.	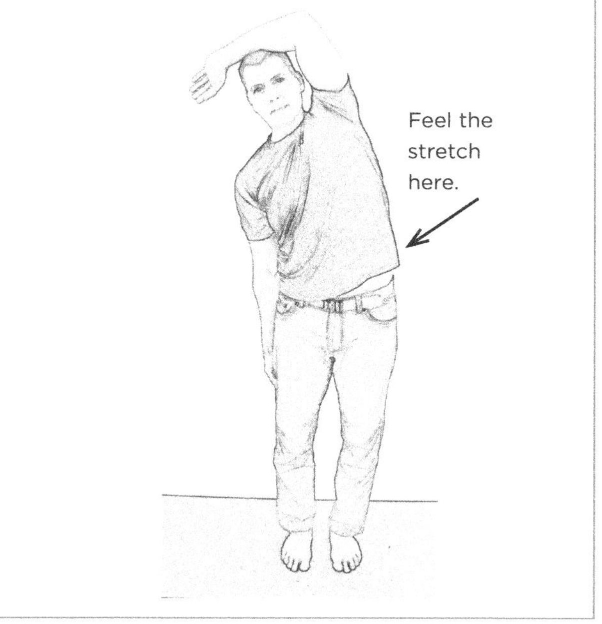

Hip Abductor Stretch	
Lie on your back. Bend one leg and place the sole of the foot on the opposite leg. Gently use your hand to pull your bent knee toward the floor. Feel the stretch on the outside of the upper leg and in the buttocks. Without letting the bent knee move, gently push the knee toward the ceiling, resisting with your hand, for five seconds. Now pull the leg into a deeper stretch toward the floor. Hold for one minute. Repeat on the other side.	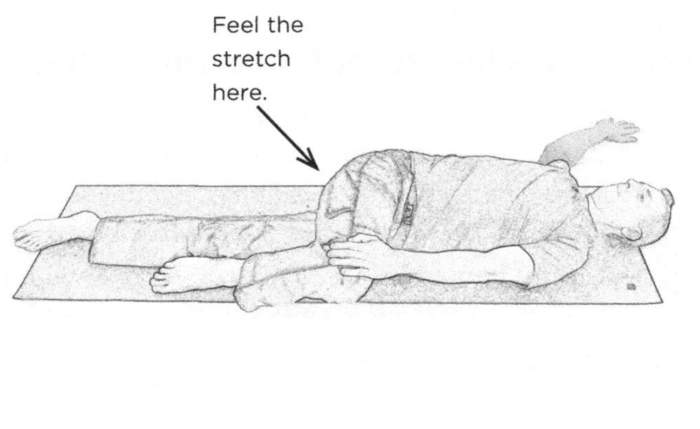

Hip Abductor Stretch (modified)	
Sit in a chair and cross one leg over the other. This will gently stretch your hip abductor muscles on the outside of the upper leg. Do not perform this exercise if your legs "fall asleep."	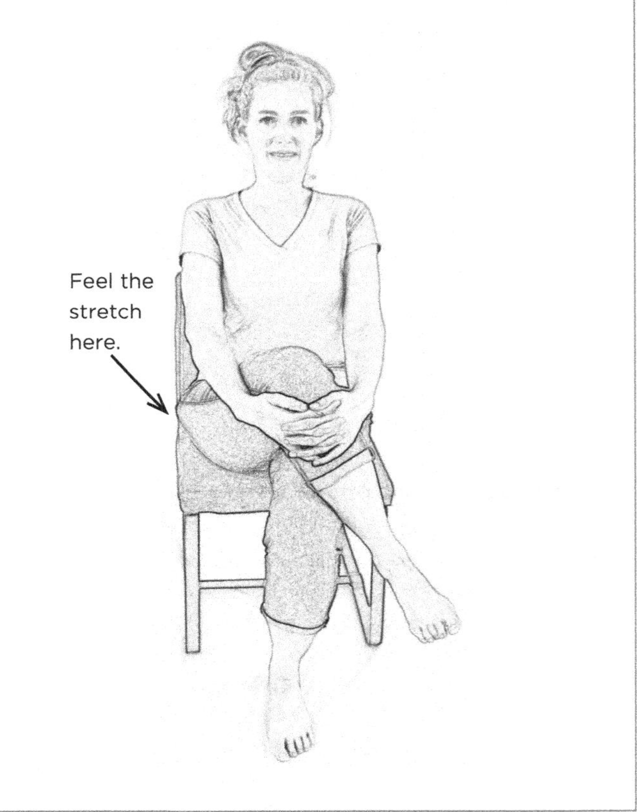

Quadriceps Stretch	
Hold onto the back of a chair or put your hand on a wall to help keep your balance. Reach back with one hand to grasp the foot and bring the heel toward the buttocks. Feel the stretch in the front of the upper leg. Push your foot gently into your hand for five seconds. Bring the heel closer to the buttocks to deepen the stretch and hold for one minute. Repeat on the other side.	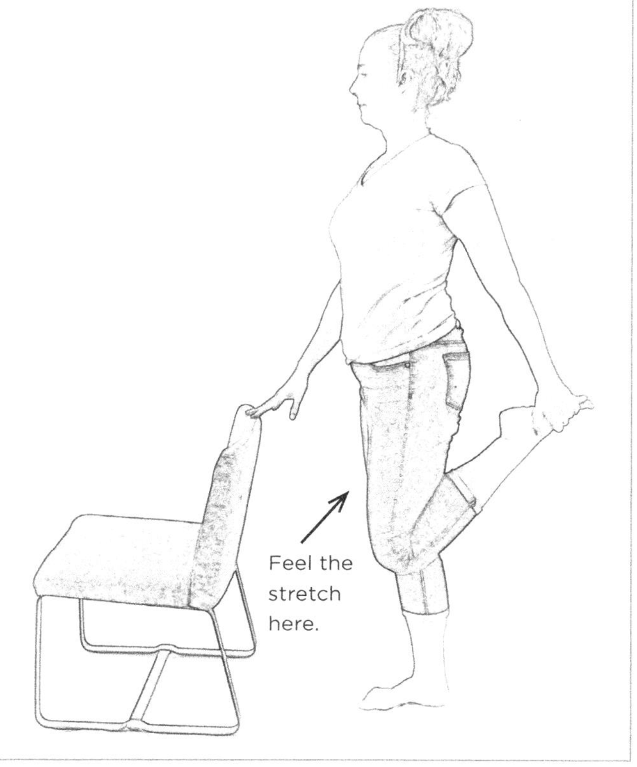

Quadriceps Stretch (modified)	
Place the top of the foot and the lower leg on a chair or sofa to achieve this stretch. Repeat on the other side.	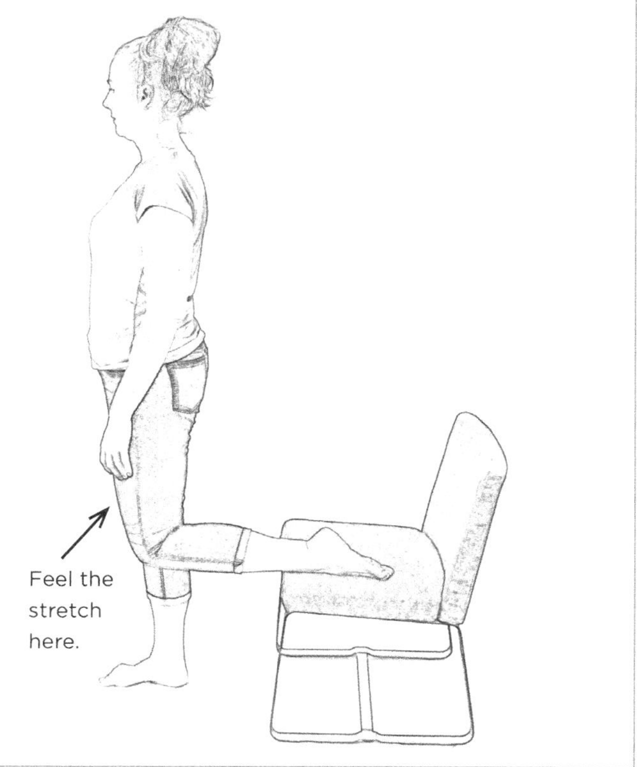

Psoas Stretch

Place one foot on a chair or stool. The foot on the floor is behind the body. Stand tall and lengthen your spine. Gently lean backward until you feel a stretch in the upper thigh. Hold for one minute. Repeat on the other side.

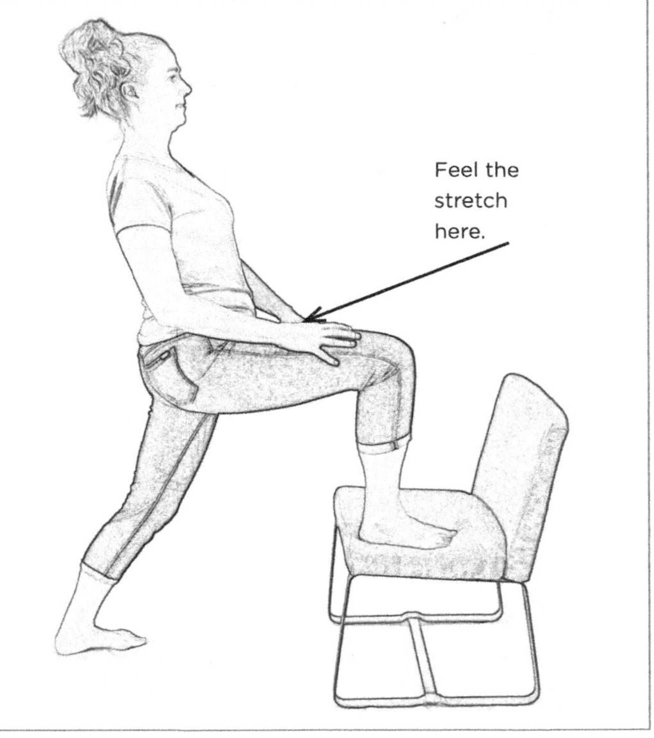

Psoas Stretch (modified)

Place your hands on your hips and gently bend backward. If this hurts the low back, you are bending back too deeply.

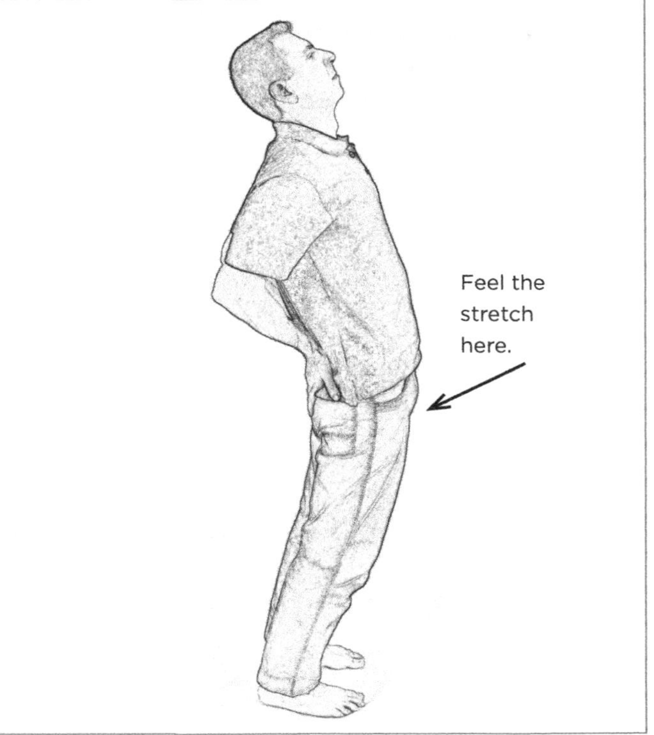

appendix c
three neck stretches

These three stretches release the muscles in the neck and bring relief to the area. They also allow increased blood flow and oxygen to the brain. Try doing these three stretches in a warm shower every morning, as the stretches work even better when the neck tissue is warm. Do these exercises one to three times a day. Always work gently and slowly.

Back of the Neck Stretch

With hands at the back of the head, pull the head forward until you feel a slight stretch. Gently push backward into your hands for five seconds, but do not let the head move. Now pull forward into a deeper stretch. Repeat a few times as long as it feels good. This will stretch the muscles along the back of your neck.

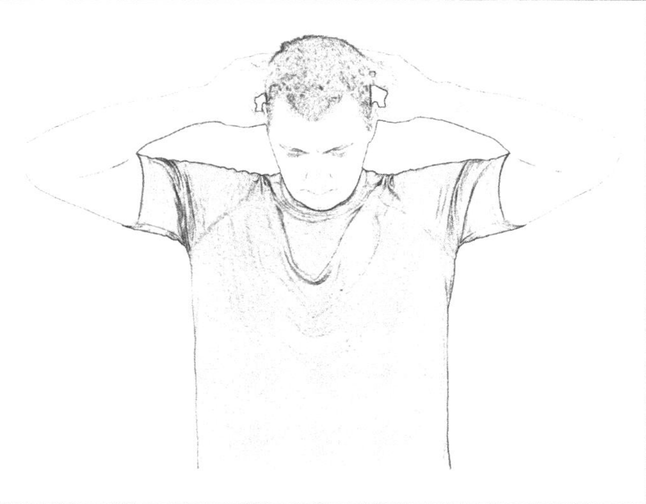

Side of the Neck Stretch

With your hand, pull your head to one side until you feel a slight stretch. Reach with the opposite hand toward the floor throughout the exercise. Gently push your head into your hand for five seconds, but do not let the head move. Now pull the head to the side into a deeper stretch. Repeat a few times as long as it feels good. Repeat on the other side. This exercise stretches the muscles on the side of your neck.

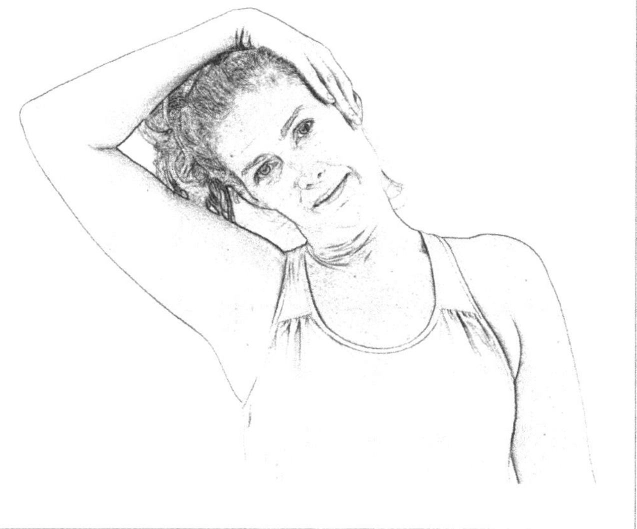

Front of the Neck Stretch	
Turn your head to one side to look over your shoulder until you feel a slight stretch in your neck. Place your hand on your cheek and gently try to turn back to the center, resisting with your hand against your cheek for five seconds. Do not let the head move. Then turn your head into a deeper stretch toward the first direction. Repeat a few times as long as it feels good. Repeat on the other side. This exercise stretches the muscles on the front of your neck.	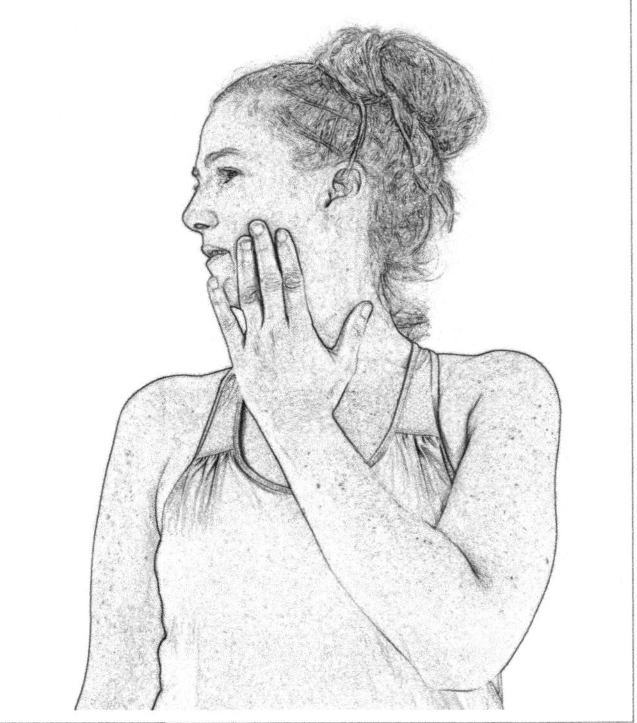

appendix d
jaw

Slacken the Jaw	
Gently push the lower jaw to one side and hold for two minutes. Repeat on the other side.	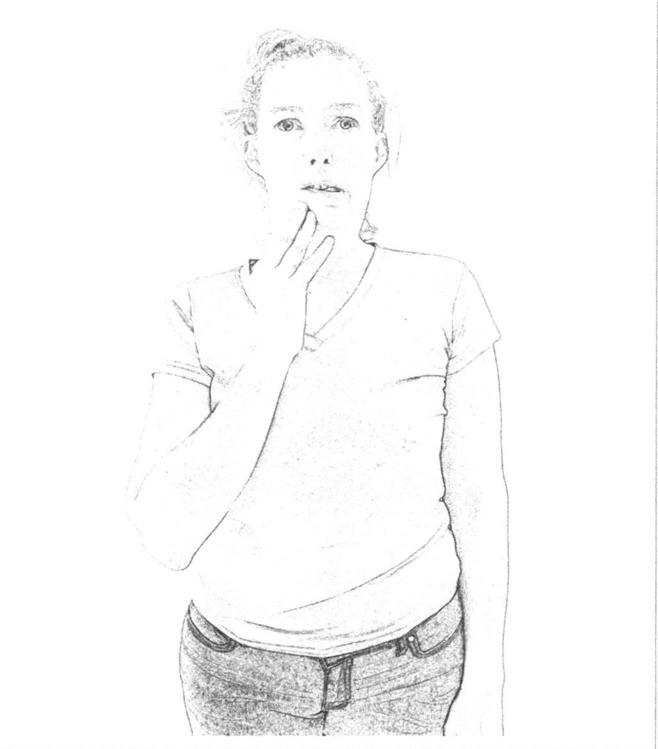

appendix e
shoulders

Shoulder Shrugs	
Gently squeeze your shoulders up toward your ears and hold for ten seconds. Repeat many times throughout the day.	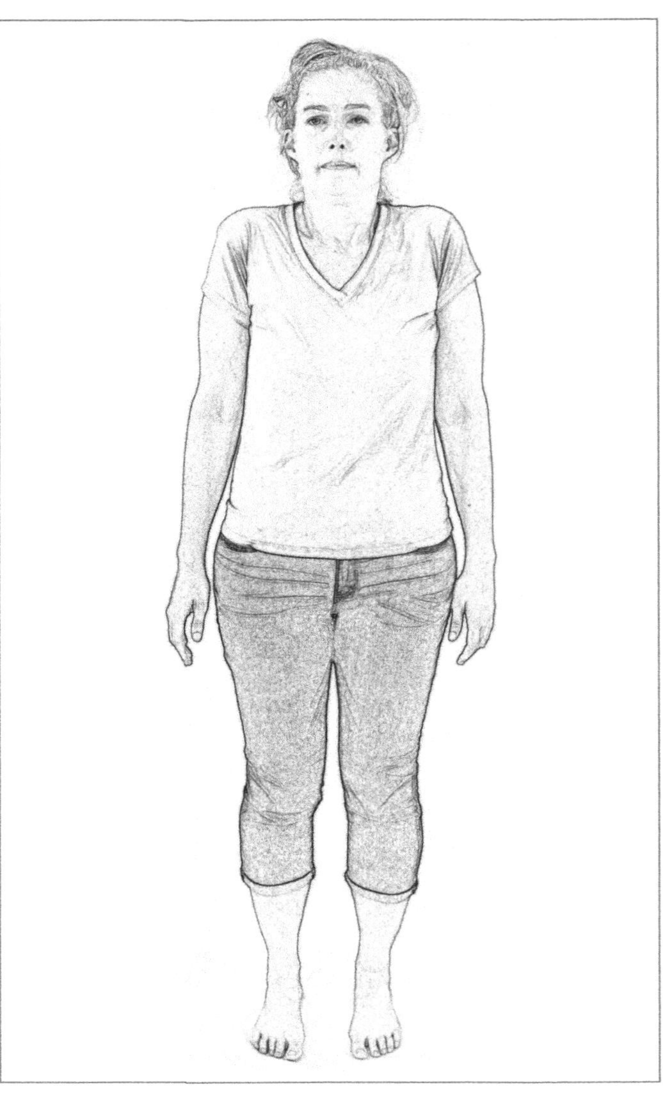

Slacken the Shoulders (Levator Scapula and Upper Trapezius)	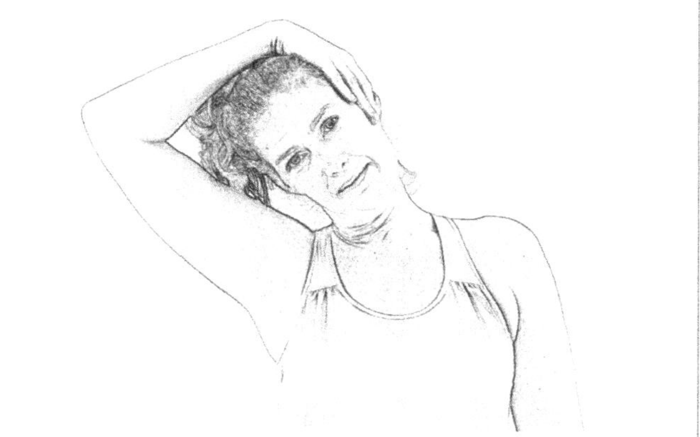
Either lying down or sitting up, place your forearm on top of the head and let it rest in that position with the head tilted toward the painful side. Hold for at least two minutes. This position will relieve tension in the shoulders, especially the upper trapezius and levator scapula. Do this anytime you feel tension in your shoulders or neck. Do not do this if it hurts to put your arm on top of your head.	

Strengthen Rhomboids & Latissimus Dorsi	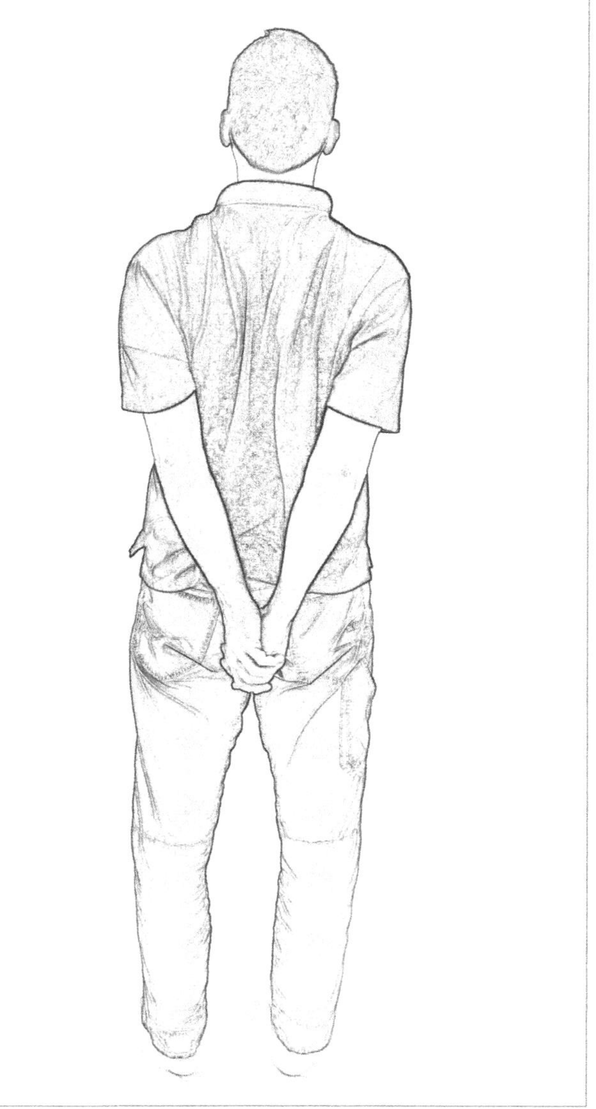
Hold your hands behind your back. Squeeze the shoulder blades together for one minute. While squeezing the shoulder blades together, also pull them down toward the floor. This will help to strengthen the muscles between the shoulder blades and the muscles below the blades, thus training the muscles to bring the head over the shoulders, improving the posture, and reducing the strain on the neck, shoulders, and upper back.	

appendix f
chest exercises

Stretch the Chest	
Squeeze shoulder blades together gently. Hold for at least two minutes. This will stretch the chest muscles and bring the shoulders back into alignment. This will release tension between the shoulder blades and the muscles known as the rhomboids.	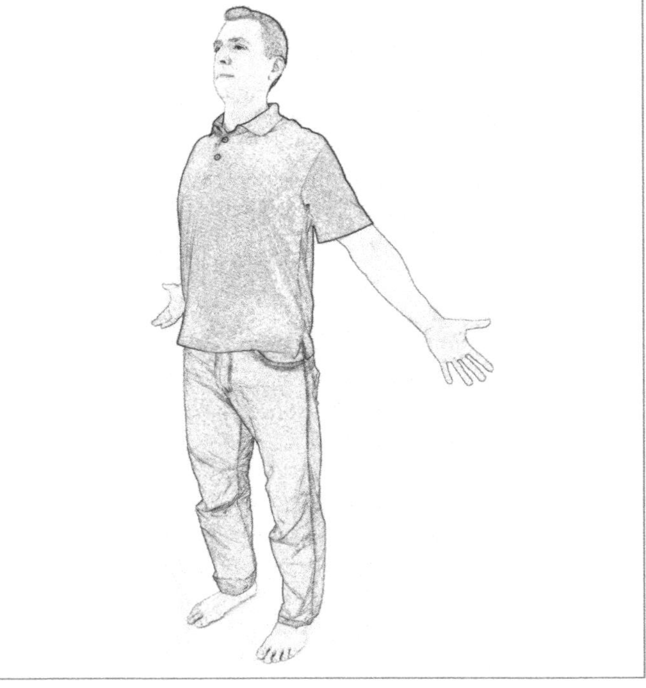

Slacken the Chest	
Place each hand on the opposite shoulder as if hugging yourself. Totally relax and hold the position for two minutes.	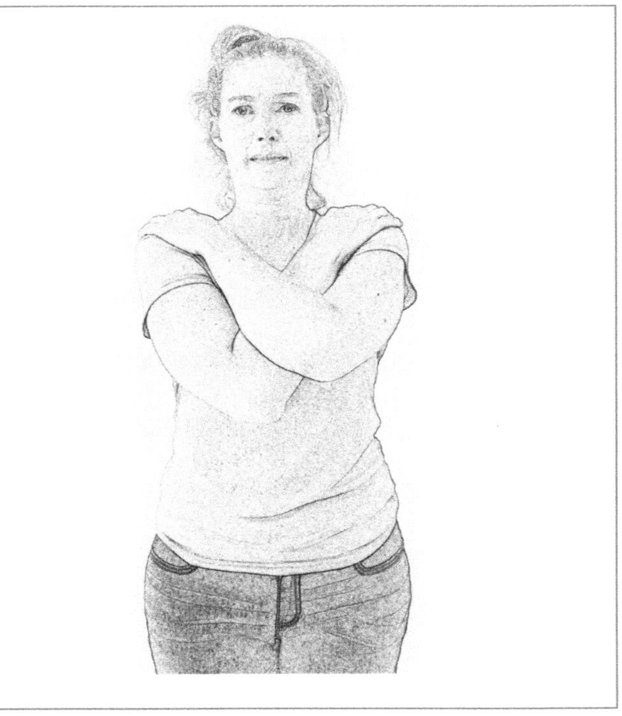

appendix g
arm and hand exercises

Elbow Tendon Release	
Gently push the tissue of the forearm toward the elbow. Hold at least two minutes.	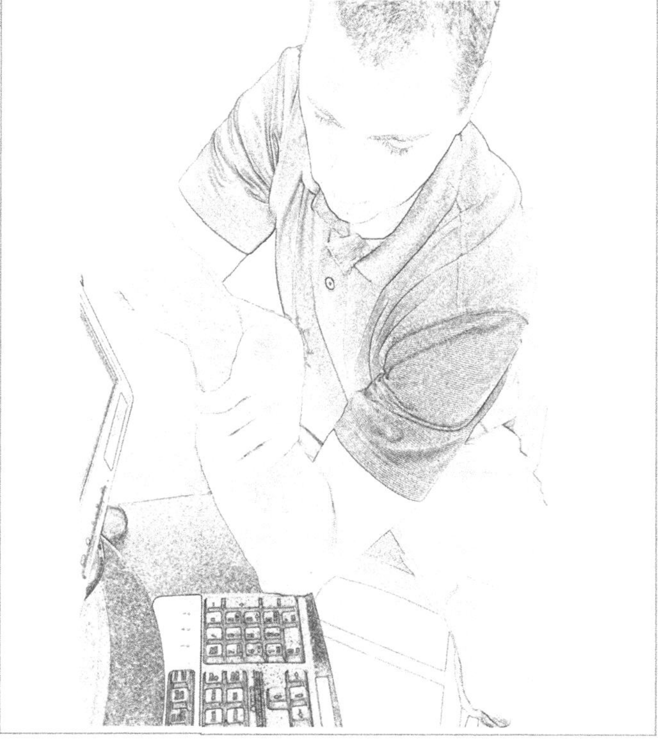

Slacken and Stretch the Forearm—two directions	
Gently twist your palm so your thumb faces down. This will release tension in your elbow and wrist. Hold at least two minutes. Then twist the arm the other way and hold for two minutes. If any of these twists bring on the symptoms, do not do these exercises until your symptoms dissipate. If you are treating carpal tunnel syndrome, keep your wrist straight. A bent wrist could bring on numbness and tingling. For tennis elbow, the wrist should be slightly bent backward. For golfer's elbow, the wrist should be slightly bent forward.	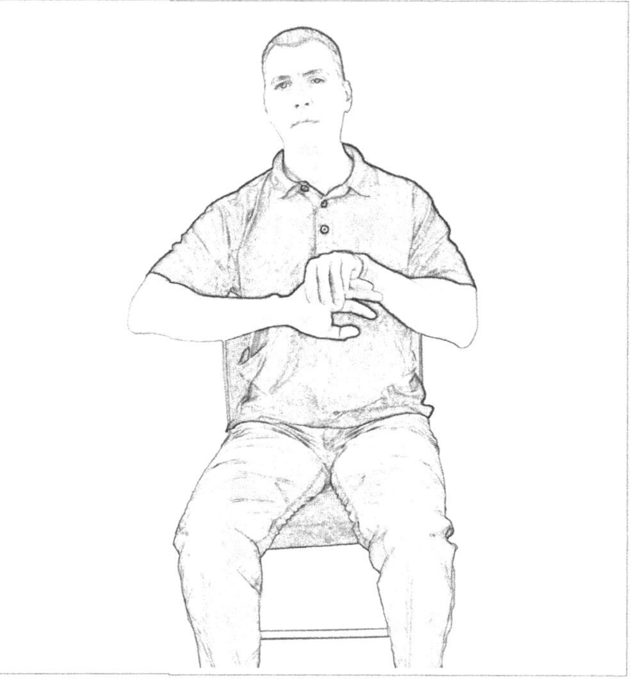

Slacken the Thumb	
Gently squeeze your thumb and palm together so that your little finger and thumb are touching. Hold at least two minutes. **If you are treating carpal tunnel syndrome, keep your wrist straight. A bent wrist could bring on numbness and tingling.**	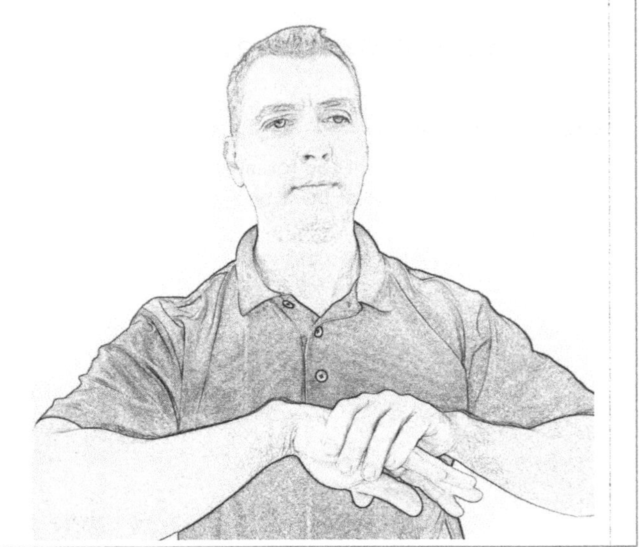

appendix h
hip and buttocks exercises

Slacken the Hip Flexors (Psoas and Quadriceps)	
Lie on your back on the floor. Bend at the hip 90 degrees and at the knees 90 degrees. Rest the lower legs on a chair or sofa. Relax in this position for at least two minutes.	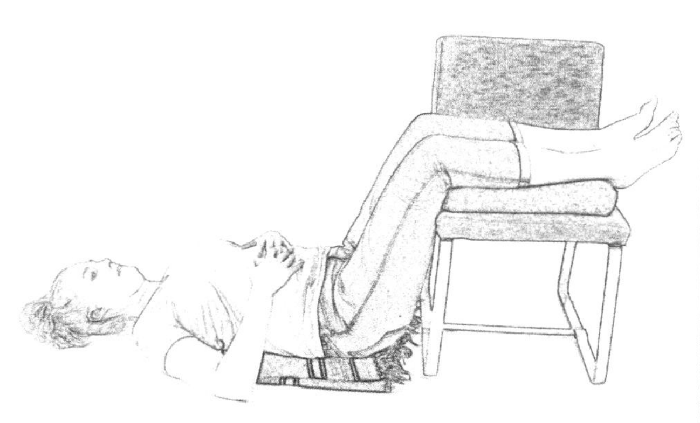

Strengthen the Hip Extensors (Hamstrings and Gluteus Maximus)	
Lie on your back on the floor. Arms are at your side. Bend your knees and keep your feet flat on the floor. Lift your hips off the floor and keep your back relatively straight. You may now clasp your hands together beneath your hips. You have the option to squeeze a block or pillow between your knees to help strengthen the adductors as well.	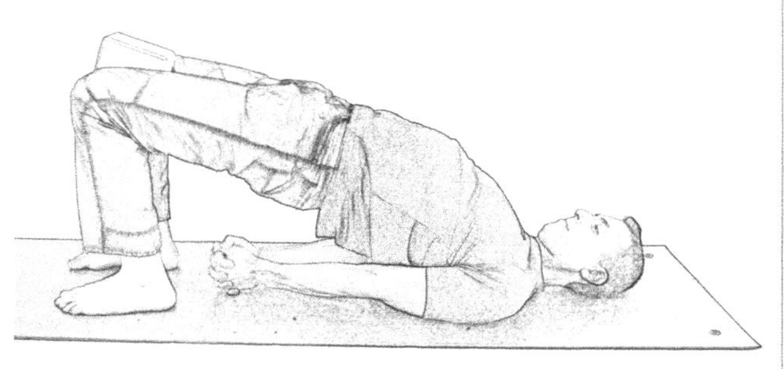

Slacken the Piriformis (Half-Frog)	
Lie on your stomach. Bend one knee and bring that leg about halfway up along the floor so that the thigh is at a right angle (or slightly less) to your torso (half-frog). Hold at least two minutes. This will release tension in your low back and the piriformis. Repeat on the other side.	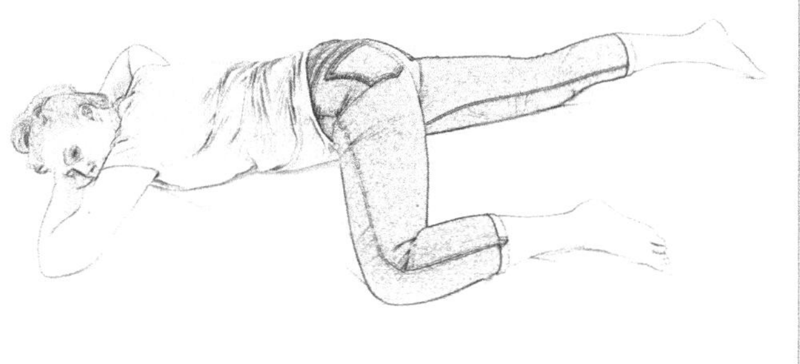

appendix i
inner thigh exercises

Slacken the Inside Thighs (Adductors)

Sit with the thighs spiraled in (pigeon-toed). Relax in this position for at least two minutes. Sitting with your legs and feet turned in will take the strain off the lower back, knees, and groin. Do not walk or stand like this; do this exercise only when sitting.

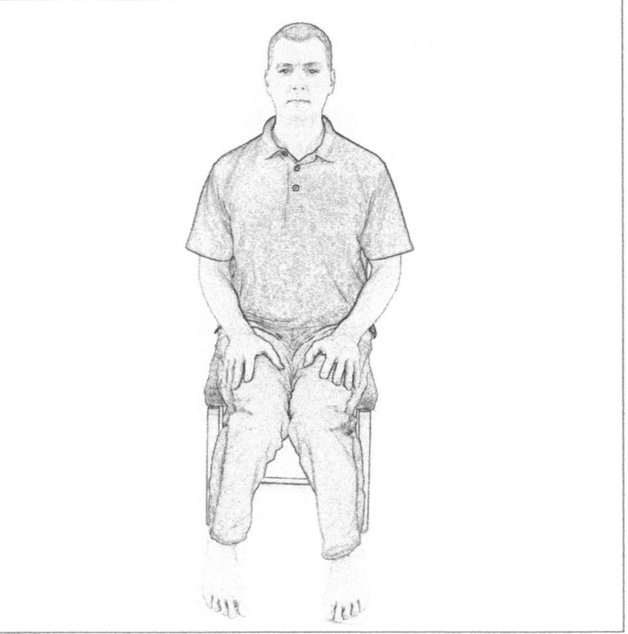

Strengthen the Inside Thighs (Adductors)

Sit in a chair. Place a pillow between the knees. You can also use a small ball. Squeeze the knees together for five seconds. Do ten of these squeezes and then rest for a minute. Do another ten squeezes and rest again for one minute. Continue in this manner until you can do five sets of ten reps. This will strengthen the muscles on the inside of your legs and begin to reduce your symptoms.

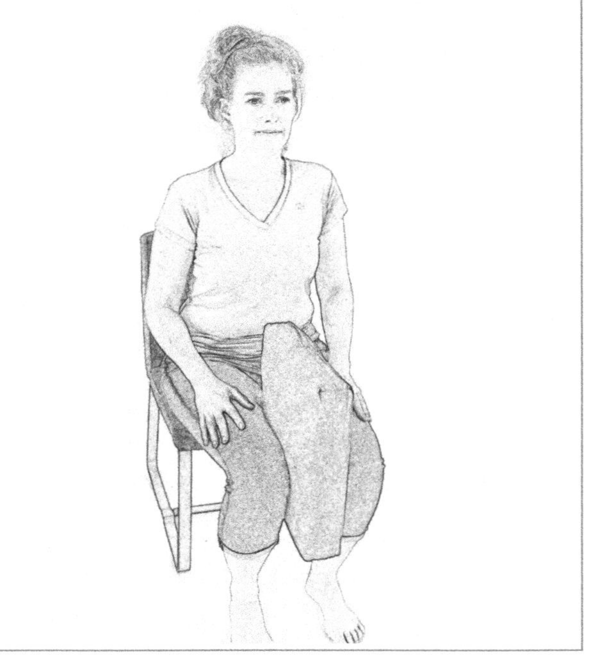

appendix j
lower leg exercises

Slacken the Calf	
Sit in a chair and place the sore foot or calf on the opposite thigh. Gently bend your foot, giving yourself a big arch. Hold that position for two minutes. This puts the calf muscle, the bottom of the foot, and the Achilles tendon into a slackened position and gives almost immediate relief. In this case, more often is better.	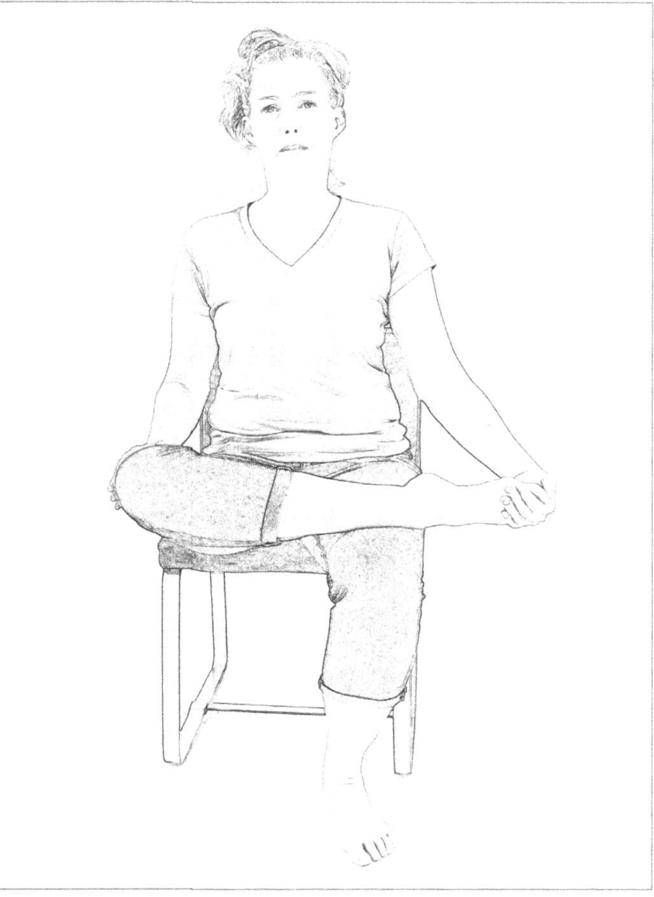

Stretch the Calf	
Stand on the edge of a step and let the heels drop gently toward the floor. Hold on to the railing. Hold for one minute. Do not stretch too deeply. If this hurts, the stretch is too deep.	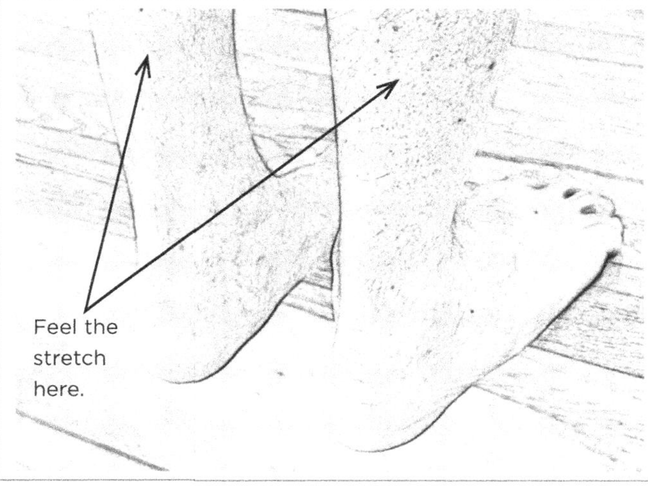

Achilles Tendon Release	
Place your foot on the opposite thigh and gently push the two ends of the tendon together. Hold for two minutes. Do this five times a day.	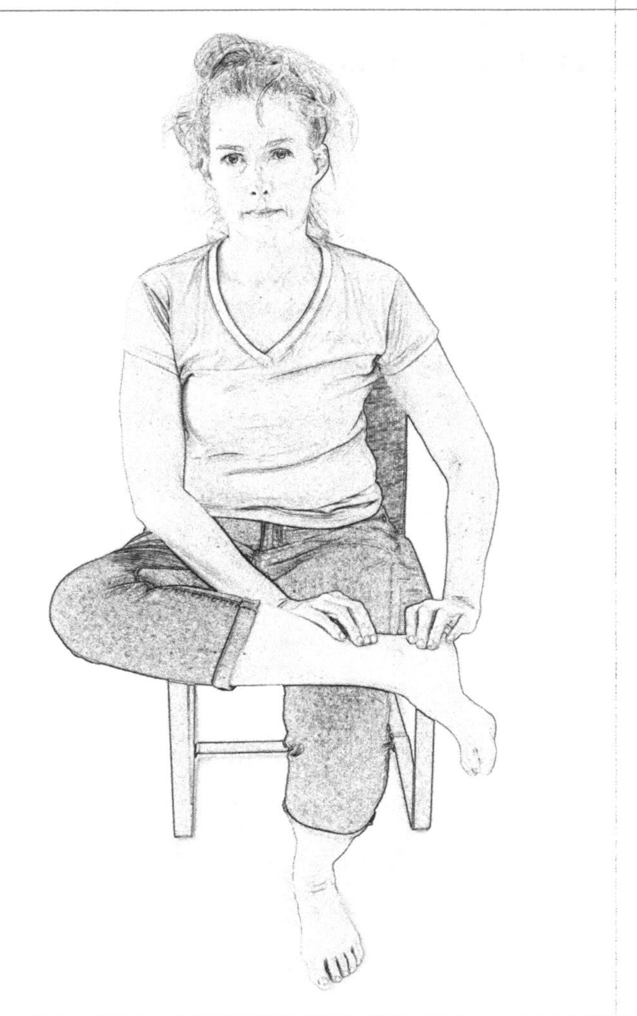

index

The page numbers for major discussions of a topic are shown in **bold** typeface. Illustrated asanas are shown by page numbers in *italic* typeface. Modified poses (e.g. modified Pigeon Pose) will be found under Pigeon Pose.

A

abdomen, 85, 122
aches, 19, 22, 27, 32–33, 35, 38, 43, 56–57, 59, 63, 67–68, 70, 92–93, 99–100, 123
Achilles tendon, 110–12, 117
activities, common, 45, 52, 58, 64–65, 70, 76, 94, 100, 106, 112, 118; daily, 26, 35, 45, 52, 58, 65, 70, 73, 76–77, 79, 82
acute, 17, 23, 27, 32–34, 56, 67, 92
adductors, long, 85–86. *See* thighs
alcohol, 38, 123
alignment, 23–24, 26–27, 29, 43–45, 50–52, 57–58, 63–64, 68–70, 87–88, 91, 93–94, 99–100, 105–6, 111–12, 117–19; neutral, 99, 106, 118
antidepressants, 119
anti-inflammatory. *See* drugs
anxiety, 42, 123, 125
arch support, 110, 112
armrests, 74, 76, 80
arms, 26, 28, 32–33, 38, 42, 44–46, 51–52, 56–58, 61–65, 67–71, 74, 76, 79–82, 115, 117
arthritis, 87, 123

B

back, 23–24, 26–29, 31–33, 36–39, 42–45, 52–53, 55–59, 63–64, 67–71, 85–88, 91–95, 97–100, 103–7, 111–12, 115–19
balance, 24–25, 27–28, 36–38, 43, 50, 56–58, 63–65, 68–71, 75, 87–88, 93–95, 99–100, 105–7, 111–12, 116–18
blood, 25, 122, 124
blood sugar, low, 43
blood vessels, 61–62
body temperature, 39
body weight, 38, 42, 124
bones, 23–24, 26, 35–36, 44, 51, 55, 57, 61, 64, 69, 91, 103, 109, 115, 117
brain, 14, 29, 38, 41, 46, 59, 63, 70, 123
brain fog, 34, 116–17, 119, 123–24
burning, 32–33, 56, 62, 67, 80, 92
bursitis. *See* pain, hip
buttocks, 33, 97-98, 100, 138-39

C

caffeine, 38, 43, 46, 116, 123
calf, 109–12, 117–18
car, 18–19, 21, 24, 26, 29, 35, 42, 59, 71, 91, 103, 121
carpal tunnel. *See* CTS
cells, 38, 41, 74, 80, 86, 92, 98, 115, 121, 123–24
cervical muscle strain. *See* pain, neck
cervical spine, 43–44, 51, 55, 57, 64, 67, 69
chair, 27–28, 32–33, 35, 68, 74, 76, 80, 87–88, 91–93, 97, 99, 103, 105, 109, 126
chemical balance, 42
chest, 33, 44–45, 51–52, 57–58, 61–62, 64, 67, 69–70, 115, 117, 122, 125

chest muscles, 27, 42, 44, 51–52, 57–58, 62, 64, 69, 71, 117
chronic, 23, 27, 29, 32–34, 56, 67, 92, 115–16, 122, 125
circulation, 46, 59, 70, 121, 124
coffee, 46–47
coldness, 32, 62
compressions, 25–26, 61–62, 94, 97, 100, 106, 111, 118
cortisone, 87, 93, 98, 105, 110
CTS (carpal tunnel syndrome), 29, 33, 79–83

D

dancing, 86, 104, 110
dehydration, 34, 41, 43, 45, 59, 70, 118, 123
depression, 119, 124
diets, 41, 116, 125; balanced, 43
discs, 25, 36, 38, 43, 55, 67, 92, 97–98, 123; problems, 45, 52, 58, 64, 70, 76, 94, 100
diuretics, 38, 46, 123–24
drugs, 22, 43, 87, 116, 127; anti-inflammatory, 26, 75, 81, 93

E

ear, 31, 49-50, 62, 144
elbows, 32, 45, 52, 58, 65, 70, 73–77, 115
elbow tendon release, 75, 147
electrolytes, 123–24
epicondylitis, 32, 73–77. *See* golfer's elbow
Epsom salt, 82, 109, 112, 118
exercises, 37–39, 43–44, 50–52, 56–57, 63–64, 68–70, 75–76, 81, 87, 93–94, 98–100, 105–6, 111, 116–18, 124–25; breathing, 42, 50, 56; daily, 124; easy-to-do-at-home, 29; forearms, 73; regular, 46, 59, 70 stretching, 27
eyes, 14, 42–43, 46, 126
eyestrain, 43

F

fascia, 25, 109; plantar, 109, 112
fatigue, 34, 42, 61, 115–16, 123
feet, 85–86, 88, 94, 99, 103–4, 106–7, 109, 111–12, 118
fibromyalgia, 29, 34, 115–19, 126
foot, 18–19, 33–34, 37, 88, 97–98, 100–101, 109–12
forearms, 28, 37, 73, 75–77, 79, 81–82
forehead, 31, 46

G

gluteal muscle group, 37
gluteus maximus, 87, 93
golfer's elbow. *See* tennis elbow
groin, 36, 85–86, 88, 92, 104, 107

H

habit, 26, 44, 51, 57, 69, 97, 117, 122
half-frog position, 93, 99–100, 105
hamstrings, 37, 87, 93
hands, 15, 18, 27–28, 32–33, 61–62, 65, 73–77, 79–83, 122, 127
headaches, 21–22, 24, 26, 29, 31, 35, 41–47, 50, 57–58, 91, 123; migraine, 21–22, 41; persistent, 31; tension, 41, 43, 45, 47
heart rate, 124–25
heat, 46, 59, 65, 70, 76, 83, 88, 94, 109, 119
heel spur, 18, 24, 26, 29, 34, 109–13
hernia, 87–88
hip, 18, 28, 33, 36–37, 85–88, 97, 103, 115
homeostasis, 27–28
hyaluronic acid injections, 105
hydrate, 38, 41, 74, 80, 86, 92, 98, 115, 123

I

ice, 76, 109
imbalances: chemical, 41, 116; hormonal, 41; muscle, habitual, 45, 52, 58, 64, 69, 75, 81, 88, 94, 100, 106, 112, 118; musculoskeletal, 27; primary pelvic, 36
inflammation, 38–39, 71, 73, 77, 86, 89, 104, 109, 113
IPT (integrated positional therapy), 14, 17, 19, 22, 27, 29, 35, 37–39
IPT wellness plan, 49-51, 53, 55-57, 59, 67-69, 71, 85, 87, 89, 103, 105, 107; for carpal tunnel syndrome, 79, 81, 83; for epicondylitis, 73, 75, 77; for fibromyalgia, 115-17, 119; for lumbar muscle strain, 91, 93, 95; for piriformis syndrome, 97, 99, 101; for plantar fasciitis, 109, 111, 113; for tension-type headaches and migraines, 41, 43, 45, 47; for thoracic outlet syndrome, 61, 63, 65

J

jaw, 31, 42, 44, 49–53
joints, 23, 36, 43, 80, 119, 123, 125; disorder, 49-51, 53; dysfunction, 39

K

knees, 14, 33–34, 36, 87–88, 94, 99, 103–7, 111, 115, 118

L

latissimus dorsi, 44, 51, 57, 64, 69
legs, 28, 33, 36, 85–86, 88, 92, 94, 97–100, 103–6, 111, 115, 118; lower, 87, 109; short, 36; upper, 36–37, 85, 88, 94, 99, 104, 106, 111, 118
levels, fitness, 124–25
lifestyle, supportive, 45, 52, 58, 64, 69, 75, 81, 88, 94, 100, 106, 112, 118
ligaments, sprained, 39
limbs, 23
lungs, 122, 126

M

medial meniscus injury. *See* pain, knee
median nerve, 79–83
medicine, Western model of, 26
meditation, 125–26
misalignment, 24–26; postural, 26
motion, 21, 24, 27, 29, 39, 74, 80, 104, 131
mouth, 31, 49–50, 122
muscle: constricted, 27; fibers, 27; groups, 42–43, 50, 57, 63, 68, 93, 99, 105, 111, 117; imbalances, 23–27, 29, 35–38, 41, 43, 61–65, 67–68, 73–76, 79–81, 85–87, 91–95, 97–100, 103–5, 109–11, 115–16; memory, 18, 28, 37; relaxants, 43, 50, 56, 62, 68, 75, 81, 93, 98, 105, 110, 116; retrain, 38; strain, 26, 41, 45, 49, 52, 55, 58, 61, 65, 70, 73, 76, 79, 85, 91; tension, 26, 41;
muscles, 24–28, 36–39, 43–44, 49–53, 57–59, 61, 63–64, 67–71, 73–75, 79–81, 85–88, 91–94, 97–100, 104–7, 117–19; adductor, 94, 99, 111, 118; forearm 73–75, 77, 79–83; long, 24, 29, 43, 50, 56, 63, 68, 75, 81, 87, 93, 99, 105, 111, 116; jaw, 49–51; masseter, 44, 51, 53; hip extensor, 87, 93; hip flexor, 37, 93, 99, 105; levator scapula, 44, 51, 57, 63, 69, 117; lumbar, 33, 91–93, 95; pectoral, short, 68; piriformis, 93, 97, 99, 105; quadriceps, 37, 93, 99, 105; scalene, 61, 63; short, 24, 29, 43, 50, 56, 63, 68, 75, 81, 87, 93, 99, 105, 111, 116; shoulder, 26, 35, 41–43; upper trapezius, 44, 51, 57, 63, 69, 117; upper trap, 46
weakness, 39

N

neck, 21, 23, 26, 28, 31–32, 35–37, 41–46, 49–53, 55–59, 61–65, 67, 69–70, 91, 115, 117–18; tight, 35, 42, 49, 55, 59, 61; strain, 43, 57, 63, 69, 93
nerve compression, 35, 56, 62, 65, 68
nerves, 25, 38, 55, 61–64, 67, 79, 92, 97–98, 101, 123
neurotransmitters, 46, 59, 70
neutral position, 85, 94, 104–5, 109, 111
numbness, 32–33, 62, 65, 79–81, 98
nutrients, 121–22

O

oxygen, 25, 44, 46, 51, 57, 59, 63, 69–70, 117, 121–22, 124

P

pain, 17–19, 21–29, 31–39, 41–47, 49–53, 55–59, 61–65, 67–71, 73–77, 85–89, 91–95, 97–101, 109–13, 115–19, 124–27; acute, 23, 34; associative, 27; chronic, 23, 29, 125; constant, 119; ear, 50; elbow, 73; foot, 36; hip, 33, 85, 87, 89, 93; knee, 103, 104, 106; localized, 27; low back, 33, 91–93, 95; lumbar, 92; muscular, 37–38, 122; musculoskeletal, 23; neck, 14, 24, 26, 29, 32, 55–59, 117; nerve, 34, 116; neuromuscular, 27; sciatic, 97–98; sensation of, 31–34, 62, 80; sharp, 71, 112; tissue, 23; unlocking, 23, 25, 27, 29; upper back, 32, 67–71
pain-free body, 24, 121
painkillers, 43, 50, 56, 62, 68, 71, 75, 81, 87, 93, 98, 105, 110, 116, 119
pain levels, reduced, 122
pain management, 27
pain medication, 106; over-the-counter, 41, 46
palm, 32-33, 147-48
pectoralis. *See* chest
pelvic tilt: anterior, 37, 93, 99, 105; forward, 45

pelvis, 36–37, 43, 49–50, 57–58, 61–65, 67–71, 85, 87–88, 91–95, 97, 99–100, 103, 105–7, 111–12, 117–18; balanced, 97; crooked, 63, 67, 71, 87, 95, 103, 109, 111; elevated, 36; rotated, 36; tilted, 36–37; unbalanced, 37, 68, 92
physical therapy, 21, 62, 68, 75, 81, 87, 93, 98, 100, 105–6, 110, 112
pillow, 126, 134, 136, 149-50
piriformis syndrome. *See* sciatica
plantar fasciitis. *See* heel spur
pollicis, 75, 81
positional therapy, 29, 35
positions, computer, 42, 45, 52, 56, 58, 64–65, 68, 70, 75–76, 81, 88, 94, 100, 106, 112; painful, 39, 131
posture, 24–26, 42, 44–46, 50–52, 55, 58, 62, 64, 91, 94, 100, 103, 106, 109, 118–19; good, 23–25, 41, 45, 55, 58, 61, 64, 70, 91, 97, 103, 115; head-forward, 42, 46, 55-56, 61, 68
practice, daily, 122, 124-26
pregnancy, 79, 98
pressure, 31, 42, 49, 62–63, 76, 80–82, 97–98, 100
protein, 43
protocols, 26, 37–39, 41, 47, 49, 53, 103, 129, 131
psoas, 36–37, 87, 93, 99, 105, 125

Q

quadriceps. *See* muscles

R

rebalancing, 38
recovery process, 74, 80, 86, 92, 98, 104, 110, 116
rehydrate, 45, 47, 59, 70, 118–19, 123–24
relief, 17, 21–22, 29, 38, 41, 71, 76, 80, 98, 109, 111, 125
reset, 18, 27–28, 37
rest, 18, 28, 37, 43, 74, 76, 80, 82, 88, 94, 100, 106, 111–12, 118
rhomboids, 27, 44, 51, 57, 64, 68–69, 117
ribs, 61, 65
running, 110, 113

S

salt, sea, 123
sciatica, 24, 26, 29, 33, 36, 97–101
shoes, improper, 110
shoulder blades, 27, 44, 51, 57, 64, 67–69, 71, 117
shoulders, 26, 28, 35–37, 41–42, 44–46, 49–52, 55, 57–59, 61–65, 67, 69–71, 91, 97, 115, 117–18; forward-rotated, 68; rounded, 44, 51, 57, 64, 69, 117
shoulder shrugs, 44, 51, 57, 63, 69
sitting, 35–36, 45–46, 56, 58, 64–65, 68, 70–71, 75, 80–81, 88, 92–95, 98–101, 104–6, 111–12, 118
skeletal components, 26
slacken, 37, 44, 51–52, 57–58, 63–64, 69, 75, 77, 79, 81, 93, 98–99, 105, 111, 117; calf, 113; shoulder, 59
sleep, 42, 79, 82, 124
slumping, 26–27, 35, 49, 91
spine, 49, 55, 65, 67, 91; crooked, 71
sports, 92, 103–4
stabbing, 32-33, 56, 67, 92
standing, 32–33, 42, 45, 56, 58, 64, 68, 70, 92, 95, 98, 110, 112
stenosis, 92; spinal, 98-99
stiffness, 32–33, 44, 51, 57, 69, 74, 115, 117
strain, 26–27, 42, 49–51, 61, 73, 85–86, 88, 91, 93–94, 99, 103–6, 109, 111, 115, 118; abnormal, 24, 137
strength, 24–25
stress, 42, 45, 49–50, 52, 55, 58, 64, 70, 75, 81, 88, 100, 103, 106, 125–27; emotional, 42, 50, 56, 126
stretch, 38–39, 43–44, 50–51, 55, 57, 62–64, 68–69, 71, 73, 97, 104–5, 111, 117–18, 125, 131; hip abductor, 86, 104; quadratus lumborum, 137; quadriceps, 139
surgery, 22, 26, 50, 56, 62–63, 68, 75, 81, 83, 87, 93, 98–99, 103, 105, 110
symptoms, 26–27, 31–34, 42–44, 50–51, 56, 62–65, 67–68, 73–76, 79–83, 86–87, 92–94, 98, 100, 104–7, 116
system: lymphatic, 45, 58, 64, 70; musculoskeletal, 23–24

T

techniques, 14, 27–28; basic muscle release, 29; muscle energy, 27
Temporomandibular Joint Disorder. *See* TMJ
tendonitis, 29, 35
tendons, 39, 73, 79–80, 85, 111, 115
tennis elbow, 24, 26, 32, 73, 77
tension, 37, 41–42, 44, 51, 57, 63, 69, 117; release, 44, 51, 57, 64, 69, 117

test, 31–34, 62, 65
therapy, 22, 29, 41
thighs, 88, 94, 99, 106–7, 111, 118, 149-50
thoracic muscle strain. *See* pain, upper back
tightness, 31–32, 42, 56, 67–68, 92, 98
tilt, posterior, 37
tingling, 32–34, 61–63, 65, 80, 98
tissues, 25–26, 37–38, 46–47, 53, 59, 70–71, 77, 79, 88, 107, 109, 119, 122
TMJ (Temporomandibular Joint Disorder), 31, 42, 49–53
TOS (thoracic outlet syndrome), 29, 32, 61–65
treatment protocols, 29, 37

V

vertebrae, 67, 123

W

walking, 17, 33–34, 36, 45–46, 58–59, 64, 70, 85–86, 104, 109–12, 124
water, 38, 46–47, 67, 74, 80, 82–83, 86, 92, 98, 104, 110, 112, 115–16, 121, 123–24; coconut, 123; intake, 38, 55, 80, 92; room temperature, 124; warm, 80, 82, 109, 112, 118
water vapor, 123
weakness, 32–33, 62, 80, 98
whiplash, 59, 62
wrist: straight, 76, 82; brace, 73, 76, 79, 82–83; extensor muscles, 73; flexor muscles, 73, 81; position, 76, 82

Y

yoga, 27, 86, 104, 107